Also by Henry Emmons, MD

The Chemistry of Joy: A Three-Step Program for Overcoming Depression through Western Science and Eastern Wisdom

The Chemistry of Calm: A Powerful, Drug-Free Plan to Quiet Your Fears and Overcome Your Anxiety

Staying Sharp

9 KEYS for a YOUTHFUL BRAIN through
MODERN SCIENCE and AGELESS WISDOM

HENRY EMMONS, MD
DAVID ALTER, PHD

Touchstone
New York   London   Toronto   Sydney   New Delhi

Touchstone
An Imprint of Simon & Schuster, Inc.
1230 Avenue of the Americas
New York, NY 10020

First Touchstone hardcover edition September 2015

TOUCHSTONE and colophon are registered trademarks of Simon & Schuster, Inc.

For information about special discounts for bulk purchases, please contact Simon & Schuster Special Sales at 1-866-506-1949 or business@simonandschuster.com.

The Simon & Schuster Speakers Bureau can bring authors to your live event. For more information or to book an event contact the Simon & Schuster Speakers Bureau at 866-248-3049 or visit our website at www.simonspeakers.com.

Interior design by Jill Putorti

Manufactured in the United States of America

10 9 8 7 6 5 4 3 2 1

Library of Congress Cataloging-in-Publication Data

Emmons, Henry.
  Staying sharp : 9 keys for a youthful brain through modern science and ancient wisdom / Henry Emmons, MD And David Alter, PhD.
      pages cm
  "A Touchstone Book."
  1. Brain—Care and hygiene. I. Alter, David. II. Title.
  QP376.E584 2015
  612.8'2—dc23
                                2015000723

ISBN 978-1-4767-5894-7
ISBN 978-1-4767-5895-4 (ebook)

Henry Emmons: To my sons, Eric and Mark, who keep me youthful, and to my wife, Jane, who keeps me real

David Alter: To my mother and father, the dual banks of love and guidance between which the current of my life continues to flow

And to Jodi, my wife, who gives that flow its energy and purpose

Contents

Part 4
The Voyage Home

- Part 1 -

The Journey Forward

You may grow old and trembling in your anatomies, you may lie awake at night listening to the disorder of your veins. . . . There is only one thing for it then—to learn. That is the only thing which the mind can never exhaust . . . never fear or distrust, and never dream of regretting.

—T. H. WHITE, *THE ONCE AND FUTURE KING*

Living a long life, a full and joyful life, requires making friends with the passing of time. It also requires a willingness to see that there is always more to discover and more to experience along the way. There is always more to learn.

As for most of us, your own life's journey may include unwanted physical and mental changes—tangible signs that you are growing older. Barely glimpsed beneath the surface, there may also be fears about what your future holds as you move beyond the expansive promise of youth.

Yet for many people, the second half of life can also be the richest and most fulfilling phase of their lives, bursting with what is yet to unfold and be discovered. It is the goal of this book to help you learn how to transform the second half of your life so that this can be true for you too.

In part 1 of *Staying Sharp*, we introduce you to the basic informa-

1

tion you'll build upon as you embark on your journey toward a well-lived life. Surprisingly, there are just three things you need to pack for this journey, but they are absolutely essential to reaching your goal.

The first of these necessities is a healthy degree of doubt. This journey demands that you courageously set aside the prevailing myths and assumptions about aging as a negative experience, as we will do in chapter 1. The second requirement is a basic understanding of the brain, which we will take up in chapter 2. There you will learn how you can rewire your brain so that it remains youthful throughout your life. Lastly, leave plenty of room in your suitcase for discovering the central role that attention plays in staying sharp. Chapter 3 will show how you can use the science of attention to dramatically improve your day-to-day experience for the rest of your life.

With your packed suitcase in hand, it is time to begin your journey. Climb aboard. While the stakes are high, it helps to remember that what you seek—what we all ultimately seek—is not so distant and is reachable by following the track we lay down. In the remainder of the book, we show you how to reach for it through nine steps to create your own path to a full and authentic life, rich with meaning and purpose. Enjoy the ride!

I'm Too Young to Feel This Old!

You Can Create a Younger Brain
and a Wiser Mind at Any Age

The Myth of Aging

Most of us can't pinpoint the exact moment we began to feel older. You know, *old* older. It creeps up on us, an accumulation of little details and changes, until one day we look around and find ourselves asking, almost daily:

Where did I put my keys again?

What's the name of that restaurant I like?

When did these stairs get so steep, anyway?

It's called a . . . wait, I know this . . . it's on the tip of my tongue . . . hang on . . . I've almost remembered it . . .

The aches and pains we might expect. But the mental lapses can be particularly unsettling. Our imaginations go to the worst possible place—*Am I losing my mind?*—and that worry can be a constant fear for those of us in midlife (and those of us who are fast approaching it).

It is easy to understand why many see aging as a bad, even frightful thing. How often have you heard someone say something like "Getting old is not for the faint of heart"? We fear the physical pain and debil-

3

ity that we so often witness, and even more so the loss of memory and mental abilities, a loss we sometimes expect as inevitable with aging.

There is a widespread notion that the brain in particular deteriorates as we age. Conventional wisdom about aging used to be some version of this:

> You are born with about 100 billion neurons. The brain's development is pretty well finished by the end of childhood. Each year after the ages of six through twelve, more and more of your brain cells die off, never to be seen again. The best you can hope for is to slow down this loss of function and try to buffer the inevitable decline of aging.

Listen when we tell you: it doesn't have to be this way! These fearful losses of function are *not* a given. Today we understand the brain in a much deeper way than ever before, and we now know how to change the brain in positive ways. For example, while it may be true that there is a loss of neurons as we get older, we now also know that the brain has stem cells that can replace some of those lost cells. In fact, the brain is remarkably resilient at repairing itself—even after something as damaging as a stroke! Neuroscience is teaching us some of the ways we can support that resilience, and we will share those findings with you throughout this book.

Yet there is more than just the hope of slowing our decline. There are ways in which aging is actually full of possibility, because our brains are *always* able to learn and our minds are continually capable of gaining wisdom. Those abilities can enhance our lives, even as we lose a few neurons along the way.

It is our premise that aging itself is neither good nor bad. We all encounter aging no matter what we do, so long as we are fortunate to live long enough. The question is not will we age, but how will we engage the aging process? In *Staying Sharp*, you'll learn techniques for facing the challenges of the second half of life with excitement instead of dread. You'll discover tools for maintaining a healthier brain, skills for enhancing wisdom, and practices that will help you live every day with a more joyful heart. Read on!

Can I Really Feel Better at This Point in My Life?

Helen's story is like so many others we hear in our practice. Now that she was in her late fifties, her brain didn't seem as sharp as it used to. She described herself as mentally "fuzzy," having trouble remembering things that she used to recall quickly and effortlessly. Her mood had been affected too, so that she was more easily frustrated and quicker to anger. A growing list of physical ailments, though none were serious, had eroded her naturally high levels of energy and optimism, leaving her feeling exhausted and depleted. She concluded her story with a statement that was part despair and part defiance: "I am more than this." Yet having tried the conventional medical routes to no avail, she'd begun to wonder, "Will I ever improve, or is this just what I have to accept as an inevitable part of aging?"

While you cannot stop yourself from aging, the good news is that the kind of decline that Helen described is neither normal nor inevitable, and you can have a lot of influence on the quality of your own aging process. Helen found that by practicing just a few of the exercises that you'll learn about in this book, she began to emerge from the mental torpor she'd found herself in. After several weeks, she felt sharper, the mental fog had lifted, and she was able to regain a sense of control and contentment in her life. It happened to Helen, and it can happen to you too.

This clarity emerges when we learn how to align ourselves with the natural way the brain is designed to work. The brain will simply express what it is in the habit of expressing. When the mind is focused with positive intentions and grows through life-affirming practices, the positive aspects of the mind that are lying dormant can evolve into new and joyful habits. *Becoming more vitally alive, feeling sharper and more mentally focused, and even awakening joy, is easier than you think.*

An East-Meets-West Approach

So how can you optimize your brain to maintain (or even further develop) your mental acuity? You can combine cutting-edge advances in neuroscience with ageless healing practices that have been keeping humans healthy for millennia. And that's where our unique backgrounds come into play.

I am Henry Emmons, MD, and I practice as an integrative (holistic) psychiatrist. As I neared the end of my medical training nearly thirty years ago, I chose to become a psychiatrist because it seemed like the natural path to understanding and embracing the whole person—body, mind, heart, and soul. But while I was leaning toward wholeness, the field of psychiatry was becoming more and more reductionist, often focused on the brain (and a few brain chemicals) to the exclusion of heart, soul, or even the rest of the body! Early in my career, I realized that practicing psychiatry in this way wasn't good for my patients or me. I had to find another way.

I was always more interested in health than disease, so I refocused my attention on what makes people healthier and happier, including the daily choices we make to care for our bodies; how we relate to our minds and their myriad thoughts and emotions; and the degree to which our hearts are alive and able to embrace all that life offers, both good and bad. This led me to study, in earnest, the fields of integrative nutrition, lifestyle medicine, ayurvedic medicine, and mindfulness practice. Neuroscience has been a natural way to tie all these disciplines together.

Over the last fifteen years, with Partners in Resilience, I have worked to weave together these disparate fields into coherent programs to help people recover from all-too-common mental health problems, without relying upon medication. My earlier books, *The Chemistry of Joy* and *The Chemistry of Calm*, describe in detail these programs for depression and anxiety, respectively. Blending Western science with Eastern wisdom, they help take the mystery out of good mental health and offer clear road maps that go beyond mere recovery from illness toward a more vital and joyful life. With *Staying Sharp*, we aim to do the same with aging—honor all aspects of what it means to be human, while blending the emerging field of neuroscience with the tried-and-true practice of mindfulness. We wish to help you not just to get by with more intact neurons but to actually grow happier and wiser as you also grow older.

And I am David Alter, PhD. I have been involved in the practice of neuropsychology and health psychology for nearly thirty years. Fifteen years ago I cofounded Partners in Healing, the holistic health center where I have explored how the brain and the mind impact health and daily functioning. I've long recognized that whole health cannot be created by a person's psychology alone. We are all mind *and* body, and my work has involved finding methods by which people can most effectively bring together these two aspects of being human to support whole health. That is why I have worked to help people develop their inner capacity to heal and grow, to use their minds to rewire their brains. My main professional goal remains assisting people to discover the paths by which their lives can become richer, more meaningful, and more purpose-driven.

My interest in translating brain science into a therapy of practical, teachable steps is a natural extension of my personal life. My mother was a teacher, my father a neurologist. From early on, the interaction between learning and brain functioning in shaping people's lives was modeled for me on a daily basis. Those interests led me to design treatment programs that combine brain-based Western learning with practical skill develop-

ment drawn from Eastern healing traditions for a wide range of conditions—migraine, chronic pain, and digestive disorders, to name a few.

While brain science has certainly shaped my personal outlook and
practice, an even more powerful influence for this book has been the
spiritual tradition in which I was raised. In a word, it taught me hope.
As Elie Wiesel, a Nobel Prize–winning author, has said, "Hope is like
peace. It is not a gift from God. It is a gift only we can give to one
another." My personal hope is that this book is our gift to you and that
through your reading and applying of the information and practices we
present, you will find renewed hope about the reward and fulfillment
that awaits you in the second half of your life.

We have worked together as a medical doctor and a neuropsychologist for more than twenty-five years, integrating the best of Western
medicine with complementary mind-body healing practices. We share
a deep commitment to helping people discover the powerful and often
underused resources they have within themselves, skills that with
practice can enable you to live a more resilient and joyful life. In *Staying Sharp* we share with you these ideas and practices that we have
been developing throughout our professional lives.

Our work is deeply rooted in the foundational advances in neuroscience of the last fifteen years. We now have a much more complete
picture of what the brain does and how it works. For example, you
may have heard of *neuroplasticity*, the brain's ability to rewire in the
face of new experience. This means that we are designed to change
and adapt throughout life—we never stop learning! New experience
prompts our brains to adjust and adapt, to create new pathways, and
we can influence the quality of and direction that those pathways take.
By the choices you make, the experiences you seek, and the skills you
cultivate through repeated practice, you are already literally rewiring
your brain. We aim to show you how to use those choices, experiences,
and skills to rewire your brain to create a more vibrant mind.

But what's truly fascinating is that the more we learn about the brain, the more validation science is giving to traditional and ancient methods of understanding how the mind works. *Mindfulness*—long a staple of Buddhist thought and practice—actually can be measured and studied using the newest brain-imaging techniques by today's neuroscientists. And *self-regulation skills* are not just important for children in the classroom; they are essential life skills that predict a child's future success and happiness as an adult. In fact, Eastern tradition and Western science are working together (and validating each other) in new, exciting ways every day. That intersection is at the center of the work we do with our patients, and it's what we will teach you in *Staying Sharp*.

With this book we aim to translate this science and wisdom into an easily understood framework you can follow to maintain and even rebuild a youthful mind, coupling these key concepts with practical and accessible steps that anyone can take at any age. These steps are especially helpful for individuals like you, who are seeking to *thrive* in the second half of life.

When Helen began to practice what we will soon teach you, she effectively tapped into the plasticity of her brain and the resilience of her mind. Neuroscience has shown us that the circuits of the brain are designed to recognize repeating patterns. And by extension, when our mind does something repeatedly, that part of the mind gets stronger. What we focus upon grows.

This inborn tendency toward pattern recognition can be refined into a positive trait: for example, we can begin to notice the many ways that our spouse, flawed though he or she may be, acts in ways that we appreciate. And sometimes we can apply our learned patterns in new ways when we encounter something new and unexpected—such as a random act of kindness by a stranger that evokes a feeling of gratitude within us—because we may be able to draw from some past experience with a similar pattern.

But the repeating of old patterns works against us, as it did for Helen, when life becomes a series of unending repetitions—"more of the same." This familiarity can lead to feelings of malaise or even mental dullness, and since so many of these patterns operate automatically and outside of our direct awareness, they can easily get in the way of personal growth.

But the story doesn't have to end there, because we are conscious beings, capable of growth through purpose and intention. The capacity for changing our brains is truly staggering. It is said that the number of possible combinations of connections among the brain's 100 billion neurons, each of which has up to ten thousand connections with other neurons, is larger than the number of atoms in the known universe!

With consistent and repeated use of the practices described in this book, Helen's neural circuits began to change for the better. By integrating the modest exercises and body-based meditations that follow, Helen felt her physical body begin to come alive with sensation. She regained a sense of being *embodied*—a whole person interconnected to a body with thoughts, feelings, sensations, and wise emotions that she could now begin to assert. She not only felt better physically; she also felt clear-headed and more mentally nimble.

Helen's story is far from unique. While your own story may contain different particulars, the avenues that she pursued are just as relevant to you. She sought connection to herself and to her life; she sought meaning and purpose; she sought pleasure and novelty; and she sought a basis of hope and belief that she could live a life that reflected the best she had to offer.

Resilient Brain, Vibrant Mind, Awakened Heart

We tend to use the words *brain* and *mind* interchangeably in our culture, but in fact they're two very different things, and they each need something different in order to age well and stay sharp. Living and aging joyfully requires three core traits that we call *resilience*, *vibrancy*, and *awakening*. *Resilience* refers to the brain, *vibrancy* deals with the mind, and *awakening* involves the heart and enables us to connect meaningfully with others.

So what is resilience? It involves the ability to keep a positive mood and a sense of well-being even in the face of significant adversity. Resilience is a result of a healthy, well-functioning brain—a youthful brain. The *capacity* for resilience is built into our brains: it is natural. But the ability to direct this capacity for resilience is a function of a vital, well-integrated, radiant mind—a vibrant mind.

We consider the brain to include the physical aspects of this pair—the anatomical structures, the physiological functions, and the chemical processes that keep us ticking. The brain is like an orchestra. When it is working well, when all the musicians are well trained, well rested, and well fed, we are *resilient*. When it is fully functioning, the brain has all the elements it needs to make rich, resonant, beautiful music. All but one, that is. You could bring together the most talented musicians with the finest instruments, but still they would not sound good without a conductor to help them come together with a beautifully coherent sound. That is the function of the mind.

The concept of mind is sometimes hard to grasp, since it is not so concrete as anatomy or chemistry. In our view, the mind serves as a guiding principle. It involves the mental, emotional, and social abilities that can generate and extend the capacity for joy. Like the conductor, it oversees the necessary attention to detail, but it doesn't get lost in it. Mind sees the big picture, and that includes the vast array of human capabilities that can transform a series of discrete notes into a symphonic work of art. Mind allows us to use our brain and body to create a life of beauty and joy.

Beautiful music can be made by a youthful brain and a vibrant mind working together in harmony. But is it still beautiful if there's no one to hear it? Doesn't music need to connect with others in order to fulfill its purpose?

That is where an awakened heart comes in. Heart involves the capacity that each of us has, whether we've used it or not, to connect deeply with others, with ourselves, and with a life full of meaning. It is through the heart that we can fully awaken to our lives and reap the benefit of having a resilient, youthful brain and a vital, vibrant mind. When the mind is conscious and the heart is awakened, we may go well beyond resilience. We may *thrive*.

As in the metaphor of the orchestra, neither brain nor mind is much good without the other. And what good would the orchestra and conductor be without an audience to enjoy them? Each and every one of us wants and needs these three elements of ourselves—a resilient brain, a vibrant mind, and an awakened heart—to be as healthy and vital as possible, to thrive for the length of our days.

In our work, we constantly encounter people like Helen who are asking some version of this essential question: *How can I live more joyfully, age more gracefully, see with more clarity, and love more deeply for the remainder of my life?* We hope that questions like this animate you as well, and we intend to explore how you might, through nine core concepts, answer them. These lessons, applied in simple ways, can help you build a resilient brain, cultivate a radiant mind, and discover an awakened heart—laying the foundations for your own joyful life.

How to Use This Book

Learning how to integrate brain, mind, and heart into a harmonious whole has never been more needed. The sheer number of demands that compete for our limited time, attention, and energy is unprecedented in human history, and it is no wonder that we cannot always manage them with ease. This pressure may partially account for the explosion of chronic health challenges that plague people the world over. And with an aging population, experts expect an epidemic of age-related brain illnesses that society will be ill equipped to confront. In the face of these challenges, developing the resilience and vitality to better adapt and thrive in the second half of life has never been more urgent.

The second half of life will no doubt be filled with unavoidable challenges. But there is a clear path through these challenges, a path rooted in brain science, in practices attentive to the physical needs of body and brain, in mindful awareness, in habits of intimacy. On this path you will move forward, despite life's hazards, toward joy.

This book is divided into four parts. Part 1 provides the background that we think will help you make more sense of the chapters that follow. Chapter 2 focuses on the structures of your brain that help you pay attention with mindful intention, while chapter 3 show us how to put that knowledge to use by describing how we can choose to apply our attention to become more present and aware.

The heart of our approach is the Staying Sharp program. This program, described in parts 2–4 of the book, consists of nine key lessons from neuroscience that together provide the key elements to growing and maintaining a youthful brain. Each chapter introduces one key lesson, with the first three keys (chapters 4–6) devoted to building a resilient brain; the next three keys (chapters 7–9) focus on cultivating a vibrant mind; and the final three keys (chapters 10–12) focus on discovering how to awaken your heart.

The Nine Keys to Staying Sharp

1. *A youthful brain loves movement.* In chapter 4, you'll learn how exercise and moving your body mindfully can directly improve brain health, energy, and the quality of your emotions.

2. *A youthful brain is well rested.* Sleep problems seem to rise exponentially as we age. In chapter 5, you'll learn how to recharge your mind through safe, natural, mind-body approaches to sleep.

3. *A youthful brain is well nourished.* In chapter 6, you'll learn about the best brain foods and supplements, as well as ways to bring mindful approaches to your eating habits.

4. *A youthful brain cultivates curiosity.* In chapter 7, we discuss the potent brain fertilizers of novelty, play, and wonder and how you can incorporate more of these into your life.

5. *A youthful brain is flexible.* In chapter 8 we will learn about neuroplasticity, the brain's amazing capacity to change and adapt through the whole of our lives. By enhancing your own ability to remain flexible, you will be able to thrive despite the challenges you will undoubtedly face in the second half of life.

6. *A youthful brain is optimistic.* While we naturally vary in degrees of optimism, it is a skill that can be honed with great rewards. In chapter 9, we highlight the science of optimism and show you how to cultivate this inner quality to enhance the legacy that you would like your life to have.

7. *A youthful brain is empathic.* Our brains are wired to care, to be generous and compassionate, and when we grow in the capacity to love well, so does our happiness. In chapter 10, we discuss the science of empathy and show how you can use it to grow in your own level of joy.

8. *A youthful brain is well connected.* We are social beings, and our brains change when we are around others. In chapter 11, we contemplate the importance of connecting with others in meaningful ways and developing an ever-growing sense of belonging in the world.

9. *A youthful brain is authentic.* Chapter 12 points us toward one of the most important goals of a well-lived life: to become more and more fully yourself. Living authentically is the fruit of all the other practices, and it can also be

its own pursuit when we develop the capacity to live consciously and fully, expressing our own deepest nature.

There is a logical progression through these stages, and we suggest that you go through the chapters in sequence. Each part builds on what has gone before, from learning to nurture the physical brain, to practicing the core mental qualities that keep the brain young and the mind vital, and finally to realizing our great human potential—to be open to life and to others, to learn to love well, and to become most fully ourselves.

You *Are* More Than This

Helen possessed hidden qualities that allowed her to gradually reclaim her life, and you have them too. She had strength. She had defiance. These qualities supported her ability to express her resilience. Even though she may have disagreed, she was not broken by her life's struggles. In fact, she stated a deeper truth when she said, "I am more than this." You too are more than this, even if you don't realize it just yet.

Each of us has an inherent resilience that can help us to engage life again. If you feel lost, as so many of us do in the middle of our lives, you may simply need some guidance to develop the skills needed to get yourself back onto the path of your own radiant life. As men who are aging ourselves, and trying to do so with some degree of grace and skill, we hope to share both what we know and how we try to live our own lives. It is possible to have a youthful, resilient brain; a vibrant, wise mind; and a joyful, awakened heart well into advanced age. That is the promise of this book.

The Brain That Time Built

How Your Brain
Became What It Is Today

It is a daunting task to build a brain.

—DAVID LINDEN

Key Concepts

- Elements of the brain of every creature that ever inhabited the earth can be found in the modern human brain.
- Different parts of the brain have developed specialized responsibilities, but it is only when they work together that people are able to reach their highest potential, particularly as we age.
- One of the keys to healthy brain functioning involves learning to apply the mental brakes before responding to an emotional or mental trigger.
- Keeping the brain well fed with stimulation, challenge, and novel experience helps the brain stay healthy well into the eighth decade of life.

Three Pounds Produce Infinite Possibilities

Isn't it strange to think that inside our skulls sits what scientists have called a "three-pound universe"—a gray and white gelatin-like object that floats in a salty sea of spinal fluid that controls every aspect of our being? Brains have been under constant construction for hundreds of millions of years, long before modern humans or even their ancient ancestors walked the earth. The modern human brain is the latest and greatest result of many grand experiments over the course of the history of all forms of life on earth.

To better understand how you can engage your mind to generate long-term vibrant health, we want to offer a simple introduction to the history and function of the modern human brain. There is no need for you to be steeped in neuroscience to appreciate what follows. By grasping some of the abilities possessed by your brain, you can begin to see how the second half of life can be a time when age, like a good wine, can ripen certain abilities to make life more joyful and fulfilling.

Our brains have billions of cells called *neurons* that form trillions of interconnections with other neurons. These interconnections create intricate and delicate electric and chemical networks in our brains, networks that are shaped by our experiences and interactions with others. And it is precisely those ongoing interactions with others that enable the brain to grow and continue to develop well into advanced age.

This amazing organ oversees and regulates even the smallest details of the moment-to-moment functions that preserve and prolong your life. Although less than 2 percent of the body's weight, the brain consumes a whopping 20 to 30 percent of its energy. If that energy is disrupted for even a moment, the result may be loss of consciousness (or worse if the blood supply isn't quickly restored). Your brain also allows you to create and express ideas. It helps you respond and react to the world around you. But most important, it is your primary organ for creating deep, loving, and lasting relationships that can fill your years with meaning and purpose.

As we age, our brains simply change. In later middle life, the brain's processing speed slows down, affecting how quickly words can be found or how rapidly new learning occurs. But the good news is that we can influence how our brain changes in specific ways, preserving some of its youthful vigor and strengthening other parts to compensate for the inevitable slowing that occurs. If we want to stay sharp and aware as we age, we ought to give our brain at least as much attention as we do our heart, skin, muscles, and other parts of the body, so that we're not frustrated—or worse, frightened—when we start to see these early signs of our brain's changing.

Is It Alzheimer's?

Brian was in his sixties when he expressed the three-word question that strikes such deep-seated fear in people moving through midlife: "Is it Alzheimer's?" Several changes in his mental abilities that he had noticed over the previous few years generated his question. For example, it was harder for him to grab the names of people, places, or events that were often frustratingly stuck "on the tip of his tongue." When talking with people in groups, he had more trouble tracking the free-flowing conversation. He found himself asking for things to be repeated more often or at other times simply allowing the conversation to go on around him while feeling like an outsider with his own peers. At other times, he noticed that he would more easily misplace a thought: he'd arrive in one room of his house only to realize he had no idea why he had just come there. What Brian didn't appreciate was how common these experiences are for people his age and older, and how often they represent changes in brain functioning that have nothing to do with the much-feared Alzheimer's disease!

Having evaluated thousands of adults in their sixties, seventies, and beyond, we've come face-to-face every day with fears like those Brian described. Aging and dying are scary prospects in our culture. The billions of dollars spent chasing promises of a fountain of youth bear witness to those fears. But what Brian expressed was an additional layer of fear that went beyond our shared mortality. He worried that if he was diagnosed with Alzheimer's disease, he would know exactly how he would die: through a slow, scary decline of mental and physical faculties. Changes to one's memory can foretell an especially dismal future, and it's a fear that many of us share.

Just when a slower, less hectic pace of life is finally on the horizon; just when the active years of raising children or building careers can begin to wind down; just when hopes for more relaxed pleasures are finally at hand, people like Brian fear that changes in their mental functioning may devastate their dreamed-of futures. He said, "It's like my own brain is betraying me."

Thankfully (and more commonly than you may suspect), Brian's question received a positive and reassuring three-word answer: "It's not Alzheimer's." His relief was palpable. Then it was replaced by appropriate questions: "If it's not Alzheimer's, then what is going on? Why are these changes occurring? What, if anything, can be done about them?"

Although Brian's fears were expressed as an either/or question— "Do I or don't I have Alzheimer's disease?"—the real issue is more subtle and needs to be identified and addressed more directly. He was really asking, "Is this the end?"

Alzheimer's is viewed as a disease for which there is no treatment and no hope. The diagnosis predicts a complete and total loss of control over one's mind and over one's future. Who among us doesn't fear that scenario?

Thankfully, as future chapters of this book will show, those assumptions are wrong on several fronts. First, even with a diagnosis of Alzheimer's disease, there are many things that can be done to maintain the quality of one's life.[1] Second, the fear of Alzheimer's often masks a whole host of fears relating to aging. *I'll become infirm. I won't be able to care for myself. I'll lose my autonomy.* The worries go on and on.

As we will show, the brain is a highly resilient and hungry organ, eager to learn and grow along with us throughout our increasingly longer life expectancy. But to assume that happens automatically is like sitting in a car and wishing it would take us where we want to go. In both cases, driving and steering are required, and the tools to help you arrive at your destination with greater vitality are within your reach.

As Brian did, we can transform fear into positive steps to put ourselves on the path to greater fulfillment. But before we learn how to heal the brain, we must first learn more about this most vital of human organs.

What Does a Healthy Brain Look Like?

How did the brain develop the form it now has? What are the basic blocks out of which it was built over countless generations? How do these brain structures impact our daily decisions, the health of our relationships, our pursuit of happiness, or our ability to rebound from life's inevitable losses? And how can we use our brain to satisfy our life's higher purposes over a nine-decade lifespan?

One way to understand the enormous complexity of the human brain is to think in terms of the layers and structures that have developed over hundreds of millions of years of evolution. There are four distinct levels of growth that reflect important stages of this development:

- the instinctive brain
- the emotional brain

- the adaptive brain
- the compassionate, social brain.

The Instinctive Brain: Our Internal Iguana

Form a fist with your hand. That fist represents the lowest and oldest of the four stages of brain development, known as the *reptilian brain*. The reptilian brain is also known as the *instinctive brain* because that's what it controls: our purest, most basic human instincts. The instinctive brain regulates basic life functions, like breathing, heart rate, resting muscle tone, and our basic metabolism; levels of arousal (such as how alert and active we are at any given moment); and the ability to recognize stimuli and respond to them quickly, determining whether something we perceive will be ignored or will elicit a rapid and automatic response. No feelings. No messy emotions. No conscious thought. No internal debates about what to do when encountering the multitude of small and large decisions we face each day.

This is the world of instinctive reaction—physical movement without conscious thought. Instincts are fast and unchanging—the same response is generated over and over in reaction to a particular stimulus. That has its advantages. For example, all of us can recall times when we agonized about some important decision we faced. Being able to act without ever laboring over those mental lists of pros and cons may seem attractive, but it would come at a price most of us wouldn't be willing to pay. It would involve a dramatically simplified brain. As Lyall Watson, a renowned scientist, once said, "If the brain were so simple we could understand it, we would be so simple we couldn't!" Lucky for us, the next layer of the human brain evolved, giving us an upgrade that affords us more options for response and gives us clear-cut advantages for survival.

The Emotional Brain:
Weaving Together Memory and Feeling

The next level upward, also known as the *limbic brain* (or the *emotional brain*), represents a big leap forward in evolutionary time. To visualize it, take your other hand and wrap it around your closed fist. This new layer of the brain contains all the old parts (the closed fist) but also new growth (the hand wrapped around the fist) that permits emotional experience and regulation. These different feeling states allow for such complex behaviors as nursing and raising our young, connecting to others in social groups, and also the ability to engage in play. (The importance of play in maintaining brain health will be described in chapter 7.) These indispensable limbic structures help make us human: they permit us to *feel*, and we can use feelings to guide us toward more complex and life-giving behaviors.

Another name for emotional experience is *affect*, which refers to a feeling state without the reflective, self-aware aspects of the experience that we usually associate with an emotion. Emotions involve sensation, but they are not one and the same. For example, the pain felt when you accidentally step on a piece of glass while walking on a beach is a *sensation*. At first, there are no emotions, no judgments, no fears—just specialized nerves in the foot that *sense* the puncture of the skin by the glass and transmit that signal up the spinal cord to the receiving centers in the reptilian brain. This is the instinctive brain (which we just learned about) in action.

What happens next shows how our brains have evolved beyond the instinctive brain to the emotional brain. When you sense the shard of glass cutting into the sole of your foot, the sensation of pain gives way almost immediately to the emotion of *fear*. This state of fear blocks out other concerns—it makes the pain/fear signal a higher priority than anything else the brain may be dealing with at the time. This is one of the key roles of emotions: they help us focus on what is most pressing and important. They help the brain decide what gets to jump to the head of the line, where it receives high priority access to the attention and energy needed to take the best action available at that particular time.

But emotion isn't the only thing our emotional brain is good at: it can also put that feeling to work in the form of motivation. Remember back to that sole of the foot that has been penetrated by the shard of glass. It is still signaling the sensation of pain, now accompanied by fear. The combination of the two quickly sends electrical signals racing to the brain via the spinal cord and creates a strong *motivational* push that leads you to hop onto your other foot and bend over to closely examine the injury.

And what if this isn't the first time you've stepped on a piece of glass? Well, that motivation will be even stronger. The *memory* of that past experience can intensify the emotional reaction and heighten the motivation and readiness to act. Memory—the ability to capture experience and store it in nerve networks for future use—was present even in the brains of primitive creatures. It offers two fundamental benefits for survival: it helps the creature remember what should be approached (like food) and what should be avoided (like predators). But having the capacity for memory was of little benefit unless it also motivated the creature to take necessary *action* related to the memory. The important evolutionary advance offered by the emotional states is to prioritize the focus of attention, tagging what is most important at any given moment. When there are so many things that compete for our attention, this ability gives a huge adaptive advantage.

Brian's fear of Alzheimer's and the dire future he imagined temporarily paralyzed him. He had been unable to shift into *action* and remain engaged in his life. Fear blotted out other possibilities and focused his mind on a negative set of beliefs that essentially said life as he knew it was over. But once the basis for that fear was sensitively but firmly discounted, he could redirect his mind to learn about things he was perfectly capable of doing to assure that his future life could be more fulfilling.

Brian used therapy sessions to explore what actions he could take. Just as important, he needed to modify his reflexive and exaggerated response to fear. As we said, when fear is powerfully activated, it grabs our attention to address the source of the fear, primarily by fighting or fleeing. Brian's learned reflex was to flee. By allowing fear to be so dominant a force in his life, he was also allowing fear to close off other more flexible, adaptive, and life-expanding possibilities. Therefore, it was important for Brian to learn to develop *distress tolerance*, or the capacity to face emotionally unsettling circumstances without being swept away by them. Chapter 3 focuses on how to place your attention where you want it to be, which is the basis for developing distress tolerance and a key component of resilience.

The emotional brain allows for coordination of emotion, motivation, and memory. But *none* of these requires any conscious self-awareness on our part. In other words, experiencing emotions, activating memories, and having motivation can all occur without any awareness that "I" am having or guiding the experience. Millions of years of evolutionary time would have to pass before such a self-conscious "I am . . ." state of mind would develop. The next stage of brain development, the adaptive brain, brought us the neocortex and helped us to become ourselves.

The Adaptive Brain: Developing Subtlety

Evolution had successfully linked the five senses—smell, taste, touch, hearing, and vision—to automatic responses driven by the instinctive brain. Next, it created a system of basic emotional states that could help us determine the most appropriate response to any particular situation: the emotional brain. What emerged next was an amazing ability to make decisions—and change our course of action—as a result of these complex emotions. This is known as *response flexibility*, and it's a hallmark of the *adaptive brain*.

Many people believe that life evolved by gradually becoming more and more complex. While the human brain is clearly more complex than the brain of a fruit fly, its complexity isn't what most distinguishes us from other animals. What makes us so special is our great ability to adjust and adapt to different environments and circumstances. This adaptive flexibility emerges as the third major stage of brain development, and it's an important resource as we move through the second half of life.

This third layer of the brain, the *neomammalian complex* (which includes the *neocortex*), sits above and around the previous two levels. The word *cortex* comes from the Latin word for "bark," which is a good description for this outer layer of the brain. Imagine your fisted hand and your other hand covering the fist, and now slipping both of them into a warm, form-fitting padded glove. That glove is the neocortex, a rich, seven-millimeter-thick layer of brain tissue that is so densely packed with nerve cells and their connections to one another that it had to begin folding in on itself as it grew larger. Otherwise, our skulls would have grown so large and heavy that our necks and shoulders wouldn't be able to hold our heads up. If laid out flat on a table, the surface area of the neocortex would cover two sheets of a city newspaper. Imagine hefting that around all day!

The folds of the neocortex created valleys (*sulci*) and ridges (*gyri*) that are divided into four main lobes, each of which assumes primary responsibility for certain types of sensory information. They are the *occipital* (processing visual information), *parietal* (processing three-dimensional spatial relationships), *temporal* (processing sounds, especially verbal language and nonverbal speech such as tone and inflection of the voice), and the *frontal* lobes (integrating and coordinating information from the other three lobes).

These four lobes take the brain's function to the next level. It is where *sensation* (ouch, glass in the foot) becomes *meaning* (next time, I'll wear shoes!). In other words, it is here that the sight, sound, touch, taste, and smell that we experience through our sense organs get integrated into a holistic experience. For example, think of a recent conversation you've had with someone while sharing a meal: the *visual* features of her face, the *sound* of her voice, and her *bodily movements* in space, the *scent* of her cologne or perfume, or the pungent *tastes* of the meal you are sharing are all fused together as one continuous and integrated experience. The neocortex weaves together the senses with social meaning for a level of processing and complexity that was simply not possible when the lower levels of the brain were running the show.

Yet there was still something missing from this amazing human brain. The challenges of living together and dealing with one another in the complex web of human relationships required the development of the fourth and final brain region.

The Compassionate, Social Brain: The Prefrontal Brain System

Brian's fear subsided when he learned that he didn't have Alzheimer's. But he still wasn't prepared to manage his fear going forward. For that to occur, Brian had to learn to use the fourth brain area—the prefrontal cortex (PFC). The PFC has five core functions upon which a compassionate and social brain can be built:

- sensing what is happening in this moment
- noticing our emotional response to what is happening

- applying the mental brakes to keep from reacting impulsively
- using memories from the past to help respond in the best possible way now
- crafting an appropriate plan and putting it into action

First, Brian learned to manage and focus attention through meditation. Then, drawing upon the PFC's five core functions, he became more attuned to his own thoughts and feelings (in his case, through self-awareness practices). With those skills, Brian was able to take a third important step forward: by becoming more emotionally vulnerable and by nurturing more positive emotions, Brian improved his relationships. By putting the brakes on his fear, he was able to turn his attention to creating a healthier self-image and more supportive connections to others.

We are wired for compassion. We are wired for connection to others. (Both these topics will be taken up in part 2.) We need to feel compassion and connection, but aging can feed a sense of increasing isolation and alienation, two aspects of age-related fear that can grow as we lose friends to illness or death.

Focusing attention, increasing tolerance for distress, and nourishing positive emotional states help us to reconnect to others. They are a fundamental antidote to isolation and loneliness. For Brian, these skills were essential to helping him not only manage fear but learn to thrive as he faced his sixties and beyond with greater optimism, eager to discover what was in store for him next.

The Lifetime of the Brain

So let's consider what happens to the brain over the course of a single lifetime. Why doesn't the brain simply become more connected and more capable as we grow older? Must we passively await the cognitive decline that seems so common in the latter decades of life?

Neuroscience researcher and author Dr. Pamela Greenwood writes, "Cognitive decline in healthy old age is neither universal nor inevitable."[2] But how do you increase the odds that you will experience a vital brain throughout *your* life? Even if decline is not inevitable, it is clear that age-related changes do occur. It is fair to ask, then, what *does* happen to the brain on the path from birth to old age?

Imagine an old forest full of mature trees that create a lush overhead canopy. The skies grow dark. A storm is coming. A lightning bolt ignites a tree, and soon a raging fire is burning through the forest, leaving the forest floor blanketed in a layer of nutrient-rich ash. The rains come, and not long after, a new forest is already emerging from the burned hulks of the old forest. Up from each acre of land will sprout nearly 15,000 new trees. But only a few of these new trees survive. By the time that forest has once again reached maturity, that number will be about 50 to 150 trees, or less than 1 percent of what was initially growing.

Over the course of our lives, our brains undergo a very similar pruning process. We are born with more neurons than we will have again at any point during the rest of our lives. Like the forest itself, most of our brain's growth occurs as a result of the active pruning of many individual neurons, while simultaneously increasing the number of connections among those that remain. In the forest, it is the density of the trees' branches that maximizes their efficiency for capturing life-giving energy from the sun. In our brain, it is the density of the interconnections among cells that maximizes the brain's ability to oversee the many life-sustaining tasks for which it is responsible.

It is worth noting that the density of these interconnections is not that different from one adult person to the next: most humans have roughly the same number of neurons. For example, Albert Einstein's brain was found to have no more connective density than that of the average person. But what *was* different about Einstein's brain was his vastly greater number of specialized brain cells, called *glial* cells, which provide the scaffolding on which the neurons grow. How glial cells enhance the ability of information to be shared within the brain isn't well understood yet.[3] It is quite clear, however, that what helped to make Einstein Einstein was the massive number and types of connecting pathways that were spread throughout his brain. The vast number of connections between his neurons and glial cells provided him many more pathways than the average person. We can't promise that you will be the next Einstein, but you can increase the *connectivity* of your brain, thereby increasing your life's vibrancy and vitality.

The particular steps you can take to increase your brain's connectivity (described in part 2) mimic the ways the brain naturally learns and grows. In that respect, our approach to vital aging cooperates with what your brain already does, which makes it easier to incorporate the steps into your life as you condition your mind and body to grow a more vibrant brain. Whether the steps we describe are *physical* (as in moving or eating), *psychological* (as in becoming more curious or seeking mental challenges), or *social* (as in deepening your connections to others with greater empathy and playfulness), they all require the same core skill set. Simply stated, they require the capacity for sustained and directed attention, the willingness to repeat the activity over and over, and an ability to mentally observe your experience without self-criticism or judgment.

The Currents of Brain Growth

As the earth's weather is generated by the ocean's currents, our own patterns of mood, perceptions, and reactions are influenced by the currents that flow within the brain. From early in life, brain growth regulates our mental and emotional nature, which is then reflected in our personality. Like the weather, our personality style is subject to change. Actively directing that change in the second half of life involves influencing the three major currents of electrical information flowing within the brain: from bottom to top; from back to front; and from right to left. By gradually shifting the direction of these currents, we can help the brain to remain refreshed and supple well into advanced age.

The *bottom-to-top* direction largely follows the path of evolution as described above, weaving instinct with the emotional, adaptive, and social brains. This bottom-up maturation of information flow takes instinctual drives and exponentially expands our range of ability so long as we have a well-functioning cortical brain.

The second direction that the brain matures is from *back to front*. The occipital, parietal, and temporal lobes of the brain feed forward sensory information to the frontal and prefrontal regions of the brain. There the information is woven together so that we can make plans and decisions based on our rich and integrated sensory experience of the world.

Perhaps the most important maturational direction occurs from *right to left*. In the first few years of life, the right side of the brain (*right hemisphere*) dominates. The right hemisphere appears to be specialized for the processing of new, never-before-encountered kinds of experiences. Over the course of a lifetime, the left hemisphere becomes more and more dominant as we accumulate experience and information and then place them into mental categories.[4]

By the time the second half of life arrives, the growing dominance of the bottom-up, back-front, and right-left shifts in the direction of electrical information flow have become very well established. With enough lived experience there is much that is familiar and much that we have mastered to help us function well in our work and our relationships, and we have a reasonable capacity to face many of life's basic day-to-day problems.

There is another important pattern that has critical implications for maintaining the vitality of the brain. The pruning of neurons that we discussed above continues throughout life, though at a much slower rate than was the case in one's first several years. In general, those areas of the brain that were the last to develop tend to be the most vulnerable to this pruning, and this can lead to cognitive decline in aging unless actions are taken to reverse these trends.

What Goes and What Grows as We Age

It was important for Brian to grasp that there are normal aspects of aging that impact neurons in the frontal and prefrontal regions. Here are some of the concerns he expressed at his initial evaluation:

- slowing of the rate at which he could process information
- diminished ability to pay attention to multiple conversations or activities at once
- more difficulty sustaining focused attention for long periods of time
- greater challenges when learning new information as compared to the past
- longer delays when retrieving information from memory (such as names, words, or directions)

These are normal, age-related changes and are not necessarily associated with disease. These mental changes mirror parallel changes that occur to the physical body (for example, slower movements, less stamina, and more difficulty learning new skills, whether that is taking up piano, swimming, or learning a foreign language). Yet we are generally more accepting of physical changes than of mental ones, perhaps because the assumption is that mental changes represent irreversible disease. We hope to change your assumptions about this.

The dorsal-lateral prefrontal cortex (DL-PFC) is the brain area most involved in problem solving, planning, and decision making. Though the last to develop, a slowing down in these abilities is often the first subtle but noticeable mental change of aging but may simply indicate normal age-related decline in this part of the brain.

A number of years ago, the saying "Use it or lose it" became quite popular. It has also proven to be quite true. Nature has a tendency to preserve *only* what is in active use and thus conserves precious energy. The bull moose grows a rack of antlers that can weigh fifty to sixty pounds. They are used primarily during the spring rut as the bulls fight with other males for the attention of and access to females. But as winter falls, lugging around fifty extra pounds is not only unproductive, it is downright dangerous. That extra weight burns up precious energy needed to survive the winter, so the moose will shed his antlers—only to grow another set next spring.

Likewise, brain networks are maintained in direct proportion to how often they are used. Any mental abilities that aren't actively used begin to degrade as the brain allots its precious resources for something else. The point is that we can take an active role in deciding which networks of the brain are going to be most actively exercised. In the process, we can increase our capacity to preserve existing abilities and delay declines in problem solving or any of the other mental functions that are important to us.

An aging brain typically follows one of two paths. If physical and mental health are maintained (the specifics of how to promote that maintenance will be the subject of later chapters), normal aging occurs with surprisingly little cognitive decline until the eighth decade of life. The other path involves diseases like Alzheimer's, which clearly and progressively damage specific structures of the brain. Over time, such illnesses produce more significant declines in cognitive health and progressively erode independent functioning.

Fears of dementia in old age seem to be growing as fast as the aging population itself. By 2020, more than 20 percent of our population will be over sixty years of age, with an increasing number of those individuals living to age eighty-five and beyond. Estimates are that for the next twenty years, ten thousand Americans will turn sixty-five every day![5]

That is a huge wave of people facing the *opportunity* to learn to age well by retaining brain vitality. Positively impacting this group's outlook on the future is especially important given that polls of baby boomers have shown that as a whole, this segment of society is more pessimistic about their future lives than any other segment of society.[6] What a loss of human potential for this group of more than 85 million people to move through the second half of their lives disconnected from the positive and enriching possibilities of healthy aging.

While we share the general concern about dementia, we believe that the statistics can be misleading. It is true that there are many more people suffering from different forms of dementia today, but that doesn't mean that dementia is "spreading" like the flu, passed along from one person to the next. Think of it this way: as more people live longer, there will be more people with dementia even if the rate at which people develop it remains the same. It will *appear* that dementia is increasing when the reality is that there are simply more older people living who may eventually develop this condition. The increased life expectancy of people in first world countries has created a serious social and medical conundrum. Our ability to extend life has galloped well ahead of our recognition of how to make those additional years reflective of a meaningful and purpose-driven life.

The brain is a voracious processor of information. It is always hungry for more, reacting in one of two ways depending on which hemisphere is doing the processing. The right hemisphere says, "Hm, that is interesting. I have never encountered that before, so let me make sense of it." The left side's response is "I recognize this. Been there, done that."

Information is either familiar because it is a recognizable pattern or it represents a new and unfamiliar pattern which must first be decoded and categorized. The right hemisphere extracts patterns from the new and unfamiliar and hands them off to the left hemisphere, which stores them for later use, and usually tags the pattern with a verbal description. Language is essential for sharing experience, as can be observed by witnessing the frustration experienced by many older adults when they can't retrieve words as quickly as they once did! With advancing age, the left hemisphere continues to serve as the storehouse of accumulated life experience, while little by little, the right hemisphere's ability to process new experience diminishes. Or does it?[7]

Does the right hemisphere age faster, leading people to become less mentally flexible, more "set in their ways"? This is a common description of older adults. Or is it that people develop daily lifestyle routines as they age that don't require them to process novel experiences? This is a classic chicken-or-egg question. The research is far from settled on this point.[8] What is known is that when people make deliberate choices to expose themselves and their brains to new and challenging experiences, like Brian learned to do, the right hemisphere shows improved functioning.

"Use it or lose it" really seems to hold true for the aging brain. What we use and stimulate persists and even grows, while what we neglect literally weakens and atrophies. A teacher once said, "Old is when your memories outnumber your dreams." This saying captures the challenge we all face as we age. Do we slip into patterns where we rest on our laurels, turning our attention more and more to where we have already been (memories), or do we continue to develop aspirations and pursue them throughout life (dreams)?

Brain Change 101

How does the aging brain differ from younger brains? There are identifiable changes in the brain's abilities, known as *cognitive faculties*, that do occur with age.[9] Detected by specialized neuropsychological tests, they fall into consistent categories. Fast processing speed remains the province of the young, no matter how well we nurture the aging brain. With each decade of life, the speed at which *new* information can be processed slows down. The ability to direct attention to multiple things at once, or to stay focused on one thing without distraction, also seems to decline with age. Working memory, which is essential for planning and reaching personal goals, becomes less efficient. With less capacity to store or use information, the ability to make more complex decisions declines with age, especially when the decisions have to be made rapidly. The braking power of the frontal and prefrontal regions can wear down too. The elderly *sometimes* show diminished ability to exercise control over emotions and actions (becoming, for example, more irritable, less patient, or more frequently depressed).

While neuropsychological tests examine what the brain is able to *do,* other types of tests, such as functional MRI or PET scans, look for changes in the physical *structure* of the brain. There is evidence that the tissues of the brain do shrink or atrophy with age. Brain imaging studies of older adults show a smaller and "leaner" brain: the actual volume of brain tissue declines with time. One area where the shrinkage is most noticeable is in the hippocampus, although thinning of the brain's cortex is also widely seen. The hippocampus is the brain structure so important for forming new memories, but one shouldn't despair. The significance of these changes remains far from clear!

While the hippocampus may shrink over time in the *average* adult, it is also the structure where the growth of new neurons (*neurogenesis*) and the sprouting of new links (*synapses*) between different neurons is most likely to occur! The shrinkage observed in the *gray matter* of the brain represents a loss of neurons—that is, a reduction in the number of brain cells. But the connections among the remaining nerve cells may become even more dense with time, like the mature trees in the forest whose branches are so dense they capture the sun's light, leaving the forest floor almost completely dark. Even studies of shrinkage of *white matter* in the brain (axons covered in fatty myelin that helps speed electrical signaling between nerve cells) don't show strong connections between the observed atrophy and cognitive decline, except in individuals clearly afflicted with dementia.[10] In spite of changes in brain *structure* with aging, there is actually very little evidence that these changes represent a loss of *functional* ability.

Moreover, when our lives are filled with stimulating mental, physical, and emotional challenges, and when those challenges don't represent negative, stressful experiences, the brain responds in very positive ways. For example, an important study found that elderly nuns who had remained quite engaged in their retirement community showed brain images suggesting considerable brain atrophy consistent with dementia. Nevertheless the nuns' daily vigorous mental activity and social interactions seemed to offer a protective benefit to each of them, since they did *not* exhibit signs of cognitive decline even into advanced old age![11]

It appears that when it comes to the brain, it isn't size that matters. It is the connections, the linkages, the chemical, electrical, and structural relationships between the billions of pieces and parts of the brain that hold the key to aging with grace and growth.

The brain is an exceptionally dynamic organ, able to adjust and adapt throughout life. Recent studies have dispelled the idea that we are born with all the brain cells we will ever have and that their number declines thereafter until death. Instead, neurogenesis continues throughout life, especially when the person maintains a stimulus-rich environment. Once formed, those new nerve cells travel (*migrate*) within the brain, following microscopic trail markers that help them arrive at their destinations, where they begin sprouting connections so they can become contributing members of more sophisticated nerve cell networks.

The old thinking was that the fatty insulation called myelin, which wraps around certain nerves to increase communication speeds from a leisurely 2 mph up to 300 mph, could never be repaired once destroyed or damaged. We now know that *new* myelin can be laid down even in old age. Therefore, even though the overall rate of processing speed may decline, the rate at which information can be shared within established brain cell networks can remain steady or even increase.

Like a tree that grows many new branches as it ages, *arborization* of new axons sprouting from a single nerve cell has been shown to occur throughout life. That may be why there can be an *inverse* relationship between brain volume and function. In other words, a *smaller* brain volume can be associated with *increased* cognitive functioning and improved mental efficiency! Think of how a seasoned musician can learn a new piece of music faster than a novice musician. The veteran's decades of musical experience have created densely interconnected circuits that link together the different areas of the brain needed to read, learn, and play the music more efficiently than the novice. Although the absolute number of neurons may be smaller, they can be massively linked to other neurons by creating many more chemical and electrical junctions—synapses—between cells. Those synaptic connections get sculpted into elegant networks that grow, adapt, and change (the process is called *neuroplastic change*) in response to the demands imposed upon them.

The aging of the brain is less sinister than many people have assumed. The dynamic capabilities of the brain are becoming better understood. More is known about how to put the brain's abilities to work to enhance the quality of the second half of life. While age may bring a slowing of mental and physical functions, the vast storehouse of experience accumulated over the course of one's life provides an important counterbalance to normal age-related declines. The strength, energy, and speed of youth are no substitute for the precious commodity we call *wisdom*. Only aging is able to bring that about, and the remainder of this book is dedicated to specific steps you can take to enhance your capacity for such wisdom.

The Power of Attention

Harnessing the Influence of the Mind to Create a Healthy Brain

The faculty of voluntarily bringing back a wandering attention, over and over again, is the very root of judgment, character, and will. . . . An education which should improve this faculty would be the education par excellence.

—WILLIAM JAMES, THE FATHER OF MODERN PSYCHOLOGY

Key Concepts

- A healthy brain is necessary, but as we age, that alone will not allow us to thrive. We also need to become more skilled at paying attention on purpose. That is, we need to cultivate *mindfulness*.
- The ability to focus attention—key to making sense of our increasingly complex world—is an art that can be learned, practiced, and refined. Being present not only makes us more effective, it also makes us happier.
- Emotional awareness, another skill that can come from a mindfulness practice, opens the gateway to a more joyful life.
- We can create a larger sense of self—that is, we can become more than we are—by intentionally cultivating higher states of being through spiritual practice.

Charles, a fifty-four-year-old midlevel manager, recounted the pressures he was under at work. He had always been a skilled worker and was well regarded by clients, but in this new era of global competition, he felt increasingly that his job was threatened. Like many corporations demanding greater efficiency and productivity, his company's increasing reliance on technology left him struggling to keep pace. "I feel like a dinosaur in a world moving faster and faster, and it's a world that I recognize less and less!" he lamented.

Such comments are heard more often now as the nature of work rapidly changes. The challenges Charles described reflect the way in which a fifty-plus-year-old brain is impacted disproportionately by the kinds of changes sweeping through the world of work early in the twenty-first century. The demands for multitasking, rapid decision making, quick adjustment to new technologies, and greater expectations place a huge burden on anyone, but especially those of us in the second half of life. To remain effective we must rely upon our ability to direct and sustain attention, and that becomes increasingly challenging as we age. To do this well requires more than a healthy brain. We also have to cultivate purposeful awareness so that we can direct our attention more skillfully.

Living in a World of Distraction

Charles provided a window into his world, and it was a world of distraction familiar by now to many of us. He spent his days on the phone, on the computer, or in meetings. But no matter what the activity, interruption was the norm.

"I keep my cell phone on vibrate, but that doesn't stop the interruptions," he said. "I'll be on the line with a client from Dallas while someone else is calling from London. Because of the time difference, I have to respond to them quickly. And then there are the texts and emails: I get dozens and dozens every day that I have to respond to. Everything is a priority, at least in someone's mind. I'm pretty good at multitasking, but I can't keep up. I can't seem to filter out the distractions!"

Charles's experience is hardly out of the ordinary. In fact, it is uncommon these days to get even one hour of truly uninterrupted, focused time. While working on your computer, you may occasionally check your Facebook page or Twitter account, receive a text or voice mail, read or respond to an email, or be interrupted by a colleague. How often are you able to complete even one memo, for example, without another message popping up and demanding your attention? Moreover, many people are now expected to be so readily available that even when they're not online, they feel as if they should be.

Is this a problem? Do such interruptions and other distractions really affect our brain's ability to focus? Aren't we capable of multitasking? With practice, can't we get better and better at rapidly shifting our attention?

The research says that such distraction makes quite a lot of difference, and we are not as good at multitasking as we think we are. In fact, most neuroscientists say that there really is no such thing as multitasking. We can't really focus on more than one thing at a time: we can just switch our attention quickly from one thing to another. And of course some people are better at that than others.

In one well-known experiment, researchers divided six young people into two teams, one dressed in black and the other in white, and they were recorded on video while tossing a basketball to one another. The video was then shown to the research subjects who were given one simple, specific task: to count how many times the team dressed in white passed the ball to their teammates.

But it wasn't their accuracy in counting that mattered to the researchers—it was whether or not they noticed the woman dressed in a gorilla costume who walked among the ball players, thumped her chest, and then wandered off the screen. Amazingly, more than half of the 192 subjects failed to notice the "gorilla in their midst"! What does this mean? The researchers' own conclusion was "that we perceive and remember only those objects and details that receive focused attention."[1]

In other words, we have to choose what to focus upon, and doing so means that we will miss a lot of other things that we deem less important at that moment. More recently, when this study was repeated with seniors over the age of sixty watching the video, the subjects were even less likely to notice the gorilla on the screen.[2] It seems that the scope of our awareness can become even more narrow as we age.

We human beings, it turns out, are not very good at attending to more than one thing at a time, but what about multitasking? Aren't we able to do more than one thing at a time?

In the 1740s, Lord Chesterfield had this to say on the matter in a letter to his son: "There is time enough for everything in the course of the day, if you do but one thing at once, but there is not time enough in the year, if you will do two things at a time." Long before we could be tempted by technology to master a torrent of information, Chesterfield espoused the virtues of a singular focus.

No matter how great the demands placed upon us, the idea of multitasking—successfully doing more than one thing at a time—seems to be a myth. The human brain can indeed quickly switch from one thing to another, but that comes at a cost. We lose time and energy when we constantly switch our focus, as Charles described in his struggles at work. Many experts say that we also become less efficient, and maybe even less intelligent, when we repeatedly shift our focus. Researchers at the University of California, Irvine, have confirmed what Charles experienced: workers may be able to compensate for task interruptions by working faster, but doing so often leads to greater stress, frustration, time pressure, and increased error rates.[3,4]

Dr. David Meyer is a psychology professor at the University of Michigan who studies multitasking. He believes that we can learn to switch tasks more effectively, but the elevation of stress hormones that result can effect short-term memory and possibly lead to more serious long-term health problems. We see this effect constantly in our own clinical practices, where the stresses of work, time pressures, and the push for productivity are among the most common causes of depression and anxiety.

Another researcher, Dr. Russell Poldrack, stated in a recent interview on National Public Radio, "We have to be aware that there is a cost to the way that our society is changing, that humans are not built to work this way. We're really built to focus. And when we sort of force ourselves to multitask, we're driving ourselves to perhaps be less efficient in the long run even though it sometimes feels like we're being more efficient."[5]

Surprisingly, those who do it the most don't become better at multitasking: they usually become *worse*. A series of experiments found that "heavy media multitaskers performed worse on a test of task-switching ability" than those who were lighter users of media, even though they were constantly practicing the very ability to switch from one task to another. The researchers concluded that this was "likely due to reduced ability to filter out interference"—that is, the subjects became less able to decide what was irrelevant and could therefore be ignored. They may have been quick to change their focus but couldn't filter out the important from the unimportant.[6]

Attention—The Gateway to the Mind

The attention management system functions as the gateway through which the brain takes in an unimaginably complex amount of information. In a single second, for example, billions of photons of light hit the light-sensitive cells of the retina. It is the brain's job to decode those electrical signals and translate them into the images we see with our eyes. At the same time we are also bombarded by sound wave information hitting our eardrums, molecules of scent upon our tongues and nostrils, and touch sensations picked up by our skin. It is a wonder we can make "sense" of all that information at all, and yet our lives literally depend upon it. It requires an unbelievably sophisticated attention management system to filter all that information, selecting the relevant signals that are buried within all the sensory background noise.

All of us have this capacity built into our brains, but as you may have noticed, not everyone is equal in their ability to direct their attention. Some people with fundamental attention problems, such as those with attention deficit disorder (ADD), may be unable to focus their attention no matter how hard they try. But even without a problem like ADD, many people have such a poor ability to manage their attention that it gets in the way of their day-to-day functioning. The struggle to pay attention has become all too common as many of us become increasingly distracted.

If you feel, like Charles, that you can't keep up or filter out the distractions, don't despair. In later chapters, we will show how you can intentionally use your mind to improve your attention, but first, let's review the elements of our complex biological system of attention. That complexity can be reduced to the four Ss: *select*, *suppress*, *sustain*, and *shift*.

- Select. With the help of the frontal region of the brain, we first have to decide what to focus on. Out of all the myriad things we *could* pay attention to, what is it that *matters most*? It is selective attention that gets us into the right mental ballpark. As an example, imagine that you open the refrigerator door with the express purpose of finding the pickle relish. There may be a hundred items in the fridge, but at that moment the only thing you're really interested in is the pickle relish. If that is where you have selectively placed your attention, you may scarcely notice anything else.

- Suppress. Because the dynamic world in which we live changes every second, the brain is constantly barraged with stimuli that compete for our attention. The ability to suppress what is *not* relevant is the partner to the ability to select what *is* relevant. It allows you, for example, to carry on a conversation despite the sound of the television in the background at a restaurant. But let's say there is a football game on the television that is also important to you—and you are facing the TV screen. Your ability to suppress may be overcome, to the chagrin of your dinner partner!

- Sustain. Without attentional staying power, we would literally jump from focus to focus to focus. We couldn't effectively plan or remember, so we would not be able to work toward our goals. In effect, we would be locked into a perpetually present moment in which such time-sensitive activities would become impossible. If you are reading this paragraph, you are using your ability to sustain attention. Otherwise your mind would drift to one of the dozens of possible distractions available to it.

- Shift. The last of the four Ss is the ability to *shift* the focus of attention, to move our attention seamlessly from one thing to another as we adapt to changing circumstances. Something new may be presented to us that at this moment we consider more important than what we'd been focused upon the moment before.

While you're talking to someone at a party, for example, it is only because your frontal region suppresses every other conversation that you are able to track the conversation you are having. Yet nearly everyone has had the experience of busily talking with one person, then suddenly turning your head to make a comment to another group about what they were just saying, as though you had been part of that conversation all along. Without realizing it, you actually *were* part of multiple conversations at the party. But your brain was tracking them at a level that *suppressed* their relevance until it picked up something of importance (say, that you were being talked about). At that instant, your brain *shifted* your focus, *selected* the direction of your attention to the new conversation, *sustained* it there long enough for you to make your comment while *suppressing* other competing stimuli, and then *shifted* back again to the person with whom you were having your original conversation.

There is indeed a staggering amount of information being filtered by the brain at any given moment, and that information directly affects our thoughts, feelings, and behaviors—whether we know it or not. Since only a tiny fraction of that information makes its way into conscious awareness, most of the time we are flying blind—operating under the direct influence of forces of which we are not even aware. Evolution has given us the brain structures we need for expanded awareness, as seen in chapter 2, but we have to effectively tap into that potential. We have to learn to channel and expand that awareness in positive directions. There is only one reliable way to do so, and that is to do it consciously—*on purpose*.

Skillfully applying attention is similar to what a good photographer can do with a quality camera—control the amount of light and depth of field by changing the size of the aperture along with the shutter speed. Similarly, we can master our own attention by learning to regulate the speed and amount of information we let in. To do this effectively, though, we have to find just the right balance between too much and too little. We have to find the middle way.

Mindfulness: Finding a New Way to Work (and Live)

There was nothing wrong with Charles (the frazzled multitasking businessman whose story we heard at the beginning of this chapter) or with his brain. He did not have ADD; he was not losing his memory; there were no problems with his attention system. He was simply overwhelmed by the sheer amount of information and the speed at which it was coming at him. He was actually very intelligent, energetic, and motivated. Yet he still struggled until he learned to allow his mind to settle and to place his attention where he chose—and to do so *consciously*, on purpose.

All of us have felt similarly overwhelmed, and we tend to respond in one of two ways. We can let in too much, becoming flooded by all the inputs coming our way. That is like the photographer who opens the aperture too wide, allowing so much light to come in that it washes out the details of the picture. That was Charles's pattern and, like him, when flooded we all become even more distractible, more ramped up with accelerated but disjointed thinking. Some of the side effects to this pattern include feeling stressed or anxious, not sleeping well, or experiencing poor memory.

The other common pattern is to shut down in a vain attempt to stop the onslaught. Then our thinking becomes slowed and we tend to feel sluggish, flat, or even a bit depressed. Like the photograph whose images are dark and shadowy, life loses its luster. Interest and motivation wane, and we settle into a state of lethargy.

In either case, we are like a novice photographer, innocently making mistakes because we are unaware that we need to regulate the aperture. Or we know that we have to regulate the light but simply lack the skill to do so. Whatever the cause, we can improve the situation by learning and practicing self-regulation, also known as the art of awareness.

Thich Nhat Hanh once said, "The most precious gift we can offer anyone is our attention." This is what is known as *mindfulness*—the ability to remain present from moment to moment on purpose, through the power of intention. It sounds simple, and it is. But there is enough subtlety and nuance to it that you could practice mindfulness your whole life and still grow in your ability to be more present. And that would be a very worthy life's pursuit!

Mindfulness is an ancient practice often associated with Buddhism.

But you don't have to be Buddhist to benefit from it, and we believe that elements of mindfulness are found in all the spiritual traditions. Over the past few decades a specific way of teaching mindfulness, known as mindfulness-based stress reduction, has become mainstream within the US health care system. We have practiced and taught it ourselves for over twenty years and have seen mindfulness classes become an important part of treatment for a host of medical and mental health problems. And for good reason—it works! The number of conditions improved with mindfulness training is indeed impressive,[7] ranging from chronic low back pain[8] to breast cancer[9] to the healthy activity of the immune system.[10,11]

The ability to focus has a lot of benefits, not the least of which is happiness. Dr. Matt Killingsworth has run an impressive survey of people's moment-to-moment happiness. He has been tracking over fifteen thousand people in all walks of life and from all over the world. He sends messages to their smartphones at random times of day and asks questions like what were they just doing at that moment, how are they feeling, and were they focused on what they were doing or were their minds wandering? Based on those self-reports, he has found that people's minds are wandering on average 47 percent of the time. Interestingly, minds wander the most when doing activities like showering or brushing the teeth (65 percent) and least when having sex (10 percent). But mind wandering pervades virtually everything we do.

So what is the connection between a wandering mind and happiness? It turns out that there is a very strong correlation; people are more likely to feel *unhappy* when their mind is *wandering*, no matter what they're doing. So even if the activity is considered unpleasant (like commuting to work) and you might think it would be nice to escape from it, people feel happier if they are present, in the moment. Mind wandering has an even stronger effect on happiness than many of the things we often think would make us happy, like how much money we make or whether we are married. And the effect seems to go in only one direction: mind wandering leads to unhappiness, but not the other way around.[12] This makes a strong case for learning to stay in the present moment more of the time, which is the essence of mindfulness.

This does not mean that we should *always* be focused and alert. The brain has likely evolved a system for being unfocused because some good can come from it. For example, a wandering mind allows for creativity and imagination, memory of the past, and planning for the future. Often our best problem solving occurs not when we're thinking hard about the problem but when we seem not to be thinking about it at all.

We can even use our tendency to wander in and out of focus as a pathway to awareness, which is essentially what happens in the age-old practice of mindfulness meditation. When first learning to meditate, one goes in and out of the present moment again and again. During meditation we *expect* our minds to wander. That is not seen as a problem. Rather, it is the repeated act of bringing ourselves back into focused awareness that strengthens our mindfulness muscles.

When our minds wander, they go into what scientists call *default mode*. That doesn't exactly mean that the brain is quiet or inactive. It just means that there is increased activity within a different network of brain areas, and this default network may actually play an important role in integrating all the information we take in. When we are focused and attentive, a very different network becomes activated. Both are necessary, both are good. But something very important seems to happen when we move intentionally from the default mode to a more focused state: we strengthen our capacity for focused awareness.

Dr. Wendy Hasenkamp is both a neuroscientist and a longtime meditator who became curious about what happens in the brain as one meditates. Her research involved functional MRI scans taken while subjects were doing a mindfulness breathing meditation. This practice involves attempting to focus on one's breath and repeatedly bringing one's focus back to the breath each time the mind has wandered off.

As soon as they became aware that their minds had wandered, the meditators pressed a button so the researchers knew about it, and then they returned their focus to the breath.

The process of moving from a wandering to a focused mind takes place in four stages: the mind wanders; you become aware that it has wandered; you shift your attention; and you sustain that attention on the object of choice—in this case the breath. This all takes about twelve seconds on average, and it happens many times during the course of a single meditation session. The MRI data showed that, indeed, different brain areas are involved with the mind-wandering versus the focused state. During the transition period, the brain goes from default mode to a focused, online mode, first by activating brain areas involved with detecting relevant events and then by putting the executive brain areas in charge. The executive areas can then keep the focus on the breath—at least for a while. This cycle of going in and out of awareness and activating the different brain systems involved appears to be good for the brain.[13]

The lesson here is that all of us repeatedly move in and out of awareness, but adding the practice of meditation offers us some real advantages. It isn't that the meditators' minds don't wander; they do. But they have become adept at *recognizing* when their minds have wandered, and that allows them to intentionally shift out of default mode and back into a focused state. Doing so engages a host of important brain areas and makes them stronger; it is like going to the gym and doing a great whole-body exercise. And like exercise, meditation is something that we can become better and better at with practice. This faculty can allow you to stay present when you need to, for example during an important meeting or conversation. It may also make you happier, as suggested by the research above, and it does so partly by freeing us from the tendency to ruminate—an activity that usually trends toward the negative. As Wendy Hasenkamp says, "Those who practice say that thoughts start to seem less 'sticky'—they don't have such a hold on you."[14]

If it feels daunting to take up a meditation practice, or if you have tried and couldn't sustain it, take heart. Research suggests that your brain can benefit from meditation more easily than you might think. One study found significant improvement in cognitive skills after practicing mindfulness meditation for *only four days* at twenty minutes per day! In this study, sixty-three student participants were divided into two groups. One group had the meditation training, and the other listened to J. R. R. Tolkien's *The Hobbit* being read aloud. Before the experiment, both groups performed equally on tests of mood, memory, attention, and vigilance. Interestingly, both groups improved in measures of their moods (perhaps *The Hobbit* is mood-altering!), but only the meditation group got better in the cognitive measures—and they performed nearly *ten times* better on a test measuring the ability to sustain focus.[15] This suggests that the ability to sustain attention may be one of the first benefits from a meditation practice, and it may not take long to achieve it. Like most good things, of course the benefits may get greater over time, but there is a lot to be said for just getting started, and some of the positive effects may show up very quickly.

Emotional Regulation— Unlocking the Capacity for Joy

If you had heard Charles talk about his work distress, you likely would have seen the same thing that we did—that he was carrying a great deal of anger and frustration. He was also scared—fearful that he might lose his job, which represented his source of income and sense of self. And somewhere beneath those emotions there was a hidden sadness, perhaps over the loss of the life he had expected to have by the age of fifty-four but didn't.

You might have sensed much of that emotion, but oddly enough Charles did not. He knew that he didn't feel good, but he could describe little beyond a vague sense of unhappiness. Like many men, he had plenty of emotions but very little awareness of them. But while men may fall into this pattern more often than women, we encounter relatively few adults of either gender who are both aware of their emotions and able to work with them in a skillful way. One's inner life can then be run by negative emotions, which none of us wants. Being aware of your emotions—and then knowing what to do with them—is an extremely helpful combination of skills known as *emotional regulation*. People who are skilled at emotional regulation tend to share a number of qualities:

- Good emotional regulators see that the full range of emotions have a role, a purpose, and a beauty all their own. All are to be honored.
- They can experience all their emotions with awareness— the pleasant, the unpleasant, and the downright awful.
- They are able to be present and enjoy their positive emotions.
- They have developed a good ability to tolerate distressing emotions.
- They can find the middle way between being flooded by emotions or suppressing them—not too much, not too little.
- They are able to stay grounded in the moment so that they don't get swept away by the really hard emotions.
- They can tune in to the emotional tone around them. Their empathy, the ability to sense what the other is feeling or needing, allows for a higher level of relationship with others.

For most of us the challenge lies not with the more pleasant or neutral emotions but with those that are difficult or unpleasant. Those challenging emotions are almost always heightened by the stress response, which activates the emotional brain, a region of the brain described in chapter 2. The stress hormones responsible for the fight-or-flight response turn up the volume of the alarm system (the *amygdala*) so that it can put the rest of the brain on high alert. That is really helpful if you are somehow in danger. Later, after the crisis abates, the memory center (the *hippocampus*) gets in the act so that we can remember to avoid a similar threat in the future.

That is all well and good if you have experienced a real threat, and if your stress system shuts off after the threat has passed. But stress in the twenty-first century has more to do with perceived threats than real ones, and as you know from your own experience, once it becomes activated, the stress system can remain on for a very long time. That tends to heighten those unpleasant emotions like anger, irritability, fear, or remorse—the very feelings that plagued Charles. If such distressing emotions are kept alive, say by going to the same stressful job five days per week, those brain centers remain in an activated state. This constant activation of distressing emotions is known as *emotional reactivity* and is one of the most common reasons for mental health problems like depression.[16] Anything that helps calm these brain centers—that lets them stand down—may not only help one feel better in the moment but also reduce the risk for chronic physical or emotional problems.

One recent study looked at participants' brain activity with fMRI (functional MRI) scans while they viewed potentially negative (distressing) pictures. Those who had been given a short course of mindfulness training were found to have less activation in their amygdala and hippocampal regions. Not only that, but the more mindful individuals required less input from the higher brain regions to have that calming effect.[17] In other words, having exercised their mindfulness muscles, they had stronger prefrontal lobes. They were then able to soothe their emotions with less effort, leaving more of their precious mental resources for other things—like toning down their stress response.

It is an apt metaphor to compare mindfulness practice to physical exercise. Eileen Luders is a researcher in the department of neurology at UCLA. She and her colleagues used a high-resolution MRI to compare the brains of twenty-two meditators and twenty-two age-matched nonmeditators. They found that the meditators actually had more gray matter (more nerve cells and neuron-to-neuron connections) in regions of the brain that are important for attention, emotion regulation, and mental flexibility. Through practice, they had grown a bigger brain, much like the sculpting of the body that happens with weight lifting. And it occurred in the brain areas that really count—specifically in the areas of the hippocampus, the orbitofrontal cortex, the thalamus, and the inferior temporal gyrus—all of which are known for regulating emotions.[18]

"We know that people who consistently meditate have a singular ability to cultivate positive emotions, retain emotional stability, and engage in mindful behavior," Luders said. "These might be the neuronal underpinnings that give meditators the outstanding ability to regulate their emotions and allow for well-adjusted responses to whatever life throws their way."[19]

Our own research corroborates such findings. At the Penny George Institute for Health and Healing in Minneapolis, Dr. Emmons developed a program based upon The Chemistry of Joy to help participants recover from depression without just relying on medication. We ran a study of forty health care professionals diagnosed with major depression. The intervention involved nutrition, movement, and mindfulness training with an emphasis on emotional regulation skills. We found "a 63–70% reduction in depression, a 48% reduction in stress, a 23% reduction in trait anxiety, and numerous improvements in quality of life, including a 52% reduction in presenteeism." (Presenteeism refers to the amount of productive work time when present in the workplace.) Those are remarkable improvements, especially when compared to treatment as usual. Even more impressive, virtually all those improvements held up for at least one year after completion of the program.[20]

Mind-body skills like meditation—the kind of skills you will learn through the rest of this book—can quiet the brain regions involved with emotional reactivity. Research suggests that meditators indeed appear to have a calmer limbic system. When you cultivate awareness, you strengthen your higher brain areas like the prefrontal cortex, which in turn can calm the emotional centers. It's like having a calm, competent parent who can gracefully soothe an upset child. And a child that learns to become skilled at managing his or her own emotional life has a much better chance of growing into a fully realized adult.

You Are More Than This—Becoming a Larger Self

After Charles had learned to calm his mind, to sharpen his focus, to experience his emotions and manage them skillfully, he was left with a few essential questions—the same sort of questions that lie beneath the surface of your life, and ours. When he got to the core of the matter, he realized that he wanted more out of whatever remained of his life. It wasn't that he wanted more money or more things or more recognition or even more love. When he slowed down enough to really examine his life, he knew that he ultimately had enough of these things. What he most wanted now was to become more fully himself.

When we confront a challenge like that—how to know ourselves, how to become more engaged with life, how to really embrace and live in harmony with who we are—we must look beyond the world of science. We cannot embark on such a journey without crossing the border from biology toward spirituality. When we do so, we are wise to look for guidance to those who have made such a journey before us.

The questions that matter most could hardly be framed more beautifully than they were by Wayne Muller in his book *How, Then, Shall We Live? Four Simple Questions That Reveal the Beauty and Meaning of Our Lives*. Trained both as a minister and a therapist, he presents us with these four explorations of life's core meaning:

- Who am I?
- What do I love?
- How shall I live, knowing I will die?
- What is my gift to the family of the Earth?

This is the stuff of spiritual practice, which we will explore more in the last section of this book. Spiritual practice can be complicated and confusing, but it needn't be. We like the way that Wayne Muller describes it: "Much of spiritual practice is just this: cutting away what must be cut, and letting remain what must remain. Knowing what to cut—this is wisdom. Being clear and strong enough to make the cut when it is time for things to go—this is courage. Together, the practices of wisdom and courage enable us, day by day and task by task, to gradually simplify our life."

What are your questions? What is your purpose in placing the power of your precious attention on this book? What is the path that you are setting off on, that we are setting off on together? Let's gather up our wisdom and courage and take the next step.

- Part 2 -

The Keys to Health

Building a Strong Foundation for a Youthful Brain

Every problem has two handles.
You can grab it by the handle of fear, or the handle of hope.
—MARGARET MITCHELL

No matter what you've heard, your brain is not destined to simply shrink or deteriorate as you age. New findings in neuroscience tell us that neuroplasticity—the capacity to create and strengthen neural pathways in the brain—continues as long as we live and breathe.

There is much that we can do to enhance this process of brain resilience. Every lifestyle choice that we make, whether it be what we eat, how we think, or whom we spend our time with, will influence the current and future state of our brains.

We can also take heart in what science is showing us about genetics: that *genetic expression* may be at least as important as the actual genes themselves. Our genetic code—our DNA—may be something we carry with us throughout our lives. But whether or not these genes become manifest in our lives depends upon many things that are affected by *how we live*. In other words, we can influence our genetic destiny through the choices we make.

When it comes to creating a youthful brain, we are not passive victims of attrition, condemned to losing precious brain cells that are never to be replaced. Recent findings show that neurogenesis, the ability to grow new brain cells from neural stem cells, continues well into your fifties, sixties—and even your eighties and nineties! This new cell growth is clearly shown to occur in the memory center, the hippocampus, which is especially encouraging if you are concerned about memory loss.

There are specific lifestyle choices we can make that influence this brain resilience, and our goal is to help you do these to the best of your ability. In the following three chapters we will guide you as you take steps to build a better, healthier, more youthful brain.

4

A Youthful Brain
Loves Movement

Key 1

Take care of your body. It's the only place you have to live.

—JIM ROHN

Key Concepts

- The body is meant to move, and failure to move is among the strongest reasons behind all the chronic health problems of the twenty-first century.
- Movement is not only exercise for the body: it is, quite literally, exercise for the brain. Movement makes the brain bigger, stronger, and faster.
- Movement protects the brain from the harmful effects of stress, and vigorous movement provides a good stress that can make you more resilient.
- It is never too late in life to reap the benefits of movement. But don't put it off any longer: start now!

Movement Is Good for
Your Body—and Your Brain

In fact, movement can act like a wonder drug for the brain. It protects brain cells from the harmful effects of oxidation; reduces inflammation throughout the body; helps normalize blood sugar; effectively treats depression; improves the ability to learn;[1] and promotes the survival of new brain cells.[2] It even helps normalize levels of the stress hormone cortisol and boosts the growth factors that can help you grow a bigger, healthier, better-connected brain.[3] Movement *is* a wonder drug!

In this chapter, we hope to discuss exercise and movement in fresh ways and to present you with new information to inspire you to add more of the miracle of movement to your life.

A few years ago, Dr. Emmons spoke to a group of Elderhostel learners. As the name suggests, this was a group of seniors. All were past retirement age, and most were over the age of seventy-five. They remained intellectually vital and were very interested in the topic of the day, which was resilience and depression. During a back-and-forth discussion about why resilience seems to be breaking down these days, Dr. Emmons suggested one possible reason: "Life is harder now than it used to be."

Yes, he really did tell an entire group of his elders that they'd had it easier in *their* day than we do now! You can imagine how that went over. Though Dr. Emmons's hair was already graying, most of the group's comments began with something like "Well, Sonny . . ." or "Young man . . ." But it was the content rather than the tone of their discussion that really left an impression.

Though they all lived in the Twin Cities at the time of this encounter, most of the elders had been raised on farms. They recalled often working six to ten hours a day, doing hard physical labor, even as children. They rightly pointed out that living on a farm in the first half of the twentieth century was anything but easy.

There are a couple of lessons to take from this story. One is not to question the hardiness of your seniors or to think that we have it harder now than our ancestors did. We don't. Another lesson is that we *humans are meant to move*, and it is only in the last couple of generations that the majority of us have become sedentary.

Just seventy to a hundred years ago, most Americans made their living through some kind of active labor, much of it agricultural. While that could be a hard life, it meant that they spent a great deal of time outdoors, got plenty of sun and fresh air, were more attuned to the seasons—and they moved their bodies for several hours per day. They may not have laced up their running shoes or lifted weights at the gym, but they moved throughout the day, just as human beings have done since the beginning of time.

By comparison, this is the minimum amount of weekly physical activity recommended for adults by the Centers for Disease Control and Prevention:

- At least 2½ hours of moderate-intensity aerobic activity per week
- OR 75 minutes of vigorous-intensity aerobic activity per week
- PLUS muscle-strengthening activity on at least 2 days per week[4]

Notice that this is a *weekly* minimum—two and a half hours per week versus six to ten hours per day of movement! Even so, the most recent government surveys tell us that only one in five adults meets even these minimum standards.[5] We're not suggesting that you go out and exercise for six hours a day. But we *are* suggesting that we think about physical activity differently. We have evolved to move. So let's think of movement in a broader way than "exercise," and let's find more ways to build it into our lives.

Our ancestors didn't have to think about this: they couldn't have avoided movement if they'd wanted to. But we *can* avoid it, and many of us do—much to the detriment of our brains. For example, recent research looked at the effects of movement on rats' brains. Half the rats got running wheels in their cages and half didn't. (There is a big difference between rats and humans: if you provide rats with a treadmill, they will actually *use* it! They ran nearly three miles per day.) After three months, the researchers injected a special dye to show any changes in a small but important part of the brain that controls the autonomic nervous system (the ANS). The ANS manages a lot of activities that we don't think about, like breathing, heart rate, and blood pressure. It is also heavily involved in the fight-or-flight stress response. If the ANS remains overactive, the stress response remains on, and that is harmful to both the brain and the heart.

They found a dramatic difference between the running and the sedentary rats. Those that ran preserved the shape and function of this crucial brain area, and their stress system remained quiet. But the brains of the sedentary group showed deterioration and they became more sensitive to the effects of stress, resulting in problems with high blood pressure and heart disease.[6]

This is the first time in human history that we have to think about movement and add it to our lives intentionally. Doing so keeps our bodies working and feeling better in nearly every way. And the benefits to the brain are nothing short of amazing!

How Does Movement Help Your Brain?

Movement Grows a Bigger Brain

There is mounting evidence that physical activity *protects* the brain. Now brain scans are showing that it can actually make your brain grow larger!

Researchers at the University of Edinburgh followed six hundred people for three years, starting at age seventy. The subjects kept detailed logs of their activities, and after three years they underwent brain scans. It was found that their brains did shrink a bit over time, but those who were sedentary lost the most brain volume, while those who remained physically active had the least amount of brain shrinkage.[7] Being active helped preserve brain size.

Another study showed that walking could increase the size of the brain's memory center. Scientists scanned the brains of 120 older adults over the course of a year. None of them were exercising regularly at the start of the study. Half the group then started an exercise program by walking for forty-five minutes a day, three days per week. The other half did not. At the end of a year, the walking group had 2 percent greater volume of the hippocampus, while the nonexercise group actually lost 1.5 percent of their brain tissue. The walking group also had better memory compared to the nonexercisers.[8] A bigger brain and better memory simply from walking three times per week—who would not want that?

Movement Makes You Happier

We work with many people who struggle with depression, anxiety, and other mood problems. It would be hard to find another physical treatment that works better or more quickly than exercise, even for rather severe depression.

A recent study looked at the impact of walking for thirty to forty-five minutes per day for five days per week. It wasn't anything strenuous—just walking at a comfortable pace. In fact, the participants got credit if they walked just 50 percent of the recommended time. The researchers wondered if this movement would help people with treatment-resistant depression, defined as lack of improvement after nine months on two or more different antidepressants. Remarkably, the walking group got better in *all* measures of depression, and most of them improved significantly. Compare that to the control group who did not add exercise: *not a single one of them improved.*[9]

Another study found that even one moderate workout can raise the mood in someone with major depression. Participants experienced a greater sense of well-being after a single thirty-minute session of walking on a treadmill—*just one session.*[10]

There are few things you can do for yourself that boost your mood as reliably as movement. Maybe that's because of chemical changes in the brain, like boosting endorphins, serotonin, or dopamine. Or maybe it's because it just feels better to be doing something that is so good for you. Either way, try it and see for yourself the power of movement to lift your mood.

Movement Protects Your Memory

Alzheimer's disease (AD) and other memory-related illnesses have become more common as the size of our population over age 65 continues to increase, and this problem is projected to get much worse. There are over 5 million Americans living with AD, and more than 40 million worldwide. The risk increases as we age: one in nine people over sixty-five have the condition, but AD afflicts nearly one third of people over eighty-five.[11] Given these numbers, and the serious consequences both to individuals and to society, the push is on to find ways to prevent it. There are medications being developed that hold promise for both prevention and treatment, but we should not ignore the power of lifestyle to protect our brains.

Researchers from UCLA conducted a Gallup poll of over 18,500 adults to assess health-related behaviors like smoking, diet, and exercise and to see if they correlated with memory problems throughout life. Surprisingly, they found that a lot of young people (ages eighteen to thirty-nine) expressed concerns about their memory. The researchers concluded that those memory issues were due to the effects of stress and multitasking rather than actual brain disease. They also found that seniors (ages sixty to ninety-nine) were the group most likely to practice healthy behaviors, and those behaviors seem to pay off. The more they chose healthy activities, including exercise, the less they expressed concerns about memory. And the impact was huge—they were up to *111 times* less likely to be worried about memory than those who did not choose the healthy behaviors.[12]

Another study, the Baltimore Longitudinal Study of Aging, looked at the fitness level of 1,400 men and women between ages nineteen and ninety-four. They used a sophisticated measure of cardiovascular fitness called the VO2 max. That is the amount of oxygen your lungs use in one minute of *strenuous* exercise: the more oxygen you use, the greater your fitness level. They took this measure on all 1,400 people and then followed them for seven years, measuring their scores on tests of memory and concentration. Sure enough, they found that being more physically fit predicted better future performance in thinking and memory.[13]

Alzheimer's disease correlates with a particular gene, known as APOE ε4. This gene is involved with the deposition of amyloid, a protein that is destructive to the brain's cortex in people with AD. Researchers followed 201 cognitively normal adults ages forty-five to eighty-eight and found that in those who carried the APOE ε4 gene, exercise helped keep this harmful protein out of their sensitive brain areas.[14] There are several other biomarkers for AD that are also improved by moderate exercise.[15]

While none of this *proves* that movement protects against Alzheimer's or memory loss, it does support the idea that movement is good for your brain. In fact, comparing all lifestyle approaches, exercise seems to have the most going for it when it comes to protecting our brains from memory problems as we age. Now if we could all just get moving!

Why Movement Works:
Fight, Flight, and Brain Fertilizer

Movement helps to keep a brain youthful in two very important ways:

- It tones down the stress response, thereby enhancing the survival of existing neurons.
- It provides brain fertilizer to improve the growth of new neurons.

Stress has been seen as the villain in much of what ails us these days, and it can indeed be quite harmful. But let's not forget that stress itself is not a bad thing. *Chronic* stress is harmful and may even put us at greater risk for many of the brain diseases associated with aging, as we will see in the next chapter. But if it is mild and short-term, stress can actually be good for us. In fact, we *need* to be stressed once in a while, and vigorous movement gives us a healthy form of stress that works to our advantage.

If you are chronically stressed out, then movement can help to diminish the harmful impact of the stress hormones. After all, the fight-or-flight response is preparing us for activity, *vigorous* activity, for moving as if our life depended upon it. When we are stressed and we *do* move vigorously, we are fulfilling our biological imperative, using up some of our stored energy and burning off the physical effects of adrenaline and cortisol. We are doing exactly what our bodies are calling us to do.

Even if you are not a chronically stressed person, your brain views exercise as a mildly stressful event—in a good way. When you choose to move, you can reap the benefits of the stress response without the potential harm that it poses. One of those benefits is that the brain makes more of the chemicals that support brain cell growth, including a protective protein called brain-derived neurotrophic factor (BDNF).

Think of BDNF as fertilizer for your brain. If you were a gardener and you placed an especially valuable new plant in the soil, you'd consider adding root starter to the soil mix. That helps the roots grow faster, farther, and more densely, giving your precious new plant a better chance to literally take root and thrive. Similarly, when you plant a new neuron in the soil of the brain, BDNF acts like root starter, influencing where new nerve roots go, pruning older, unnecessary nerve branches, and creating denser, richer neuronal networks. It even helps nerve cells connect with one another, ensuring their survival and enhancing their role in the function of the all-important neural circuits.[16]

Many brain diseases, including depression and anxiety,[17] Alzheimer's,[18] and Parkinson's disease,[19] have been linked to low levels of BDNF. The protein protects the brain from the harmful effects of cortisol, so when BDNF is deficient, neurons are less likely to survive the onslaught of stress. Coupled with a diminished ability to create new brain cells, this loss of neurons may explain how stress shrinks the hippocampus—something we want to avoid at all costs in order to preserve memory as we age.[20]

Movement is one of the most potent ways to elevate levels of BDNF and create greater production of new cells, as demonstrated by the research on mice that were allowed to run on a treadmill. The running mice had *twice as many* new neurons as those that remained sedentary, and they had more branching roots that were better prepared to connect with other neurons.[21] Moreover, the benefits of exercise on BDNF began within just a few days and lasted for several weeks and movement was just as effective for older mice as it was for the young.[22,23]

It is good to become stressed once in a while, especially if you do so voluntarily through occasional vigorous exercise. But if you don't like to exercise, or you can't exercise vigorously, take heart. As we'll describe below, moving your body even modestly can protect you from stress, anxiety, depression, and age-related decline. Movement can give you a more youthful brain. So whether you move fast or slow, with vigor or ease, you will still reap the benefits—so long as you move.

It's Never Too Late, but Start *Now*

It makes sense that if you remain active, you are likely to experience less physical and mental decline. But what if you've been, shall we say, reticent about exercise throughout your life? And now later in life you think, *It's too late. I've rolled the dice and now there's not much I can do.* If you have been something of a couch potato your whole life, can you still get the protective benefits of exercise?

It appears that you can. A 2009 study in the *British Medical Journal* found that men who had been sedentary until they turned fifty, but who then increased their activity level, showed the same improvement in lifespan as those who had been active throughout their lives.[24] Please understand that we are not suggesting that you wait until you turn fifty (or later) to become active! But it is truly never too late to start. So if you are not active now, start immediately.

If you're thinking, *I'll be more active after I retire,* think again. On the surface, it seems as if you could move more often after retiring because of the extra time you free up by not working forty hours or more each week. But a recent study in England puts that notion into question. The researchers followed 3,334 people for several years and asked about things like physical activity and TV viewing. The participants, ranging in age from forty-five to seventy-nine, were all working when they entered the study, but one quarter of them had retired by the end of the study. Researchers found that activity levels actually *declined*—significantly—after retirement. [25]

If you are already a regular exerciser, don't ever stop. And if you are not yet moving, then start right now—no matter how long it's been, and no matter your age. So long as you start slowly and do it safely, it is always good to move! Here's how.

Symphony for a Youthful Brain: Three Movements and a Coda

Remember, it is *movement* that we want to encourage, not merely *exercise*. Let's compare physical activity to a musical composition in three parts. As in a symphony, each of the three movements is self-contained. They can be performed separately and still be lovely and valuable. But when performed in sequence, they build on one another, revealing the symphony's full beauty and power.

Likewise, you can choose to do any one of the following forms of movement, and it will do good things for your brain. And if you really want to ensure a youthful brain, do all of them. You don't have to do them perfectly, and of course you can choose other activities, ones that appeal to you more than the ones we suggest. So long as you move, and do it as often and as consistently as you can, you will be building a better brain. Your future self will thank you.

The First Movement: Andante

The term *andante* literally means "at a walking pace." This first and most essential aspect of movement can be summarized in two words: *just move*. In this section, we want to encourage intentional movement: movement that is purposeful, frequent, repetitive, and integrated into your daily life. We will focus on two very simple, very accessible types of movement: standing and walking.

Everyone, regardless of age or current level of activity, can benefit by these and all of the recommendations that follow. But of course if you have been sedentary, you must begin adding activity safely and slowly.

◇◇

Be sure to be guided by your physician regarding how to start and how quickly to increase your activity levels, especially if you have any of the following:

- a known heart condition
- chest discomfort with or without physical exertion
- loss of balance due to dizziness
- loss of consciousness
- joint problems
- medication for high blood pressure or heart problems
- any other reason to avoid physical activity

(Source: *Physical Activity Readiness Questionnaire* or PAR-Q, developed by the British Columbia Ministry of Health)

◇◇

Don't Just Sit There—Stand Up!

We can safely say that few of us are moving several hours per day, as our ancestors did. And according to government statistics, only one in five of us is exercising the recommended two and a half hours per week. What are we doing the rest of the time? Mostly sitting.

Dr. Joan Vernikos was previously the director of NASA's Life Sciences Division, and part of her job was to keep astronauts healthy. She's written a book based on her experience called *Sitting Kills, Moving Heals*, where she makes the point that sitting for prolonged periods is quite unhealthy, even if you are fit and otherwise exercise regularly.

It was observed years ago that astronauts (who are generally in great shape) appeared to age prematurely while in space for prolonged periods of time. Like a patient confined to bed rest, they lost muscle mass very quickly. The problem, it seems, had to do with lack of movement against gravity.

We need to constantly interact with gravity and engage our large postural muscles to maintain healthy functional movement, muscle tone, and flexibility. The simplest way to do that is to stand up from a sitting position. That's really all there is to it—just stand up! You don't need to keep standing. You just need to stand up frequently.

The key is not how *many times* you stand up, but rather how *often* you stand up over the whole course of your day. It is far more beneficial, Dr. Vernikos says, to stand once every few minutes throughout the day than it is to stand up many times in quick succession. Doing thirty squats in a row may seem more worthwhile because it feels like *exercise*, but you get far more benefit by standing up thirty times spread out over the course of the day. In this case, recurrent movement clearly trumps concentrated bursts of exercise.

- If you sit for long periods during your workday, try to shift your position often. It may help to sit on an exercise ball or to use a simple upright chair without armrests or a stool without a back.
- Stand up several times per hour (every fifteen to twenty minutes) throughout the day. Set a timer if you need to.
- Do a couple of slow squats if you like before sitting down again. Or get up and reach for a book off the shelf or a cup from the counter. Or pick something up off the floor.
- Organize your office so that you have to get up for things like the phone, printer, or files. At home, put away your TV remote so that you have to get up to change the channel (or just put away your TV).

Walking—There Is No Better Movement

The best way for most of us to add more movement in our lives is to walk. It doesn't have to be a fitness walk, though that is good too. Any kind of walking will do—getting a drink at the water cooler, running an errand, taking a leisurely stroll in the park. It is inexpensive, takes little skill or training, is safe, and is almost always available. Walking strengthens all the major muscle groups, improves bone density, and as we showed earlier, can grow a bigger brain, boost mood, and preserve memory. If you're not inclined to go to the gym for exercise, then walking is *the* activity for you.

How to Walk

- Walk tall and upright rather than leaning forward. Keep your buttocks tucked in so that you slightly flatten the arch in your back. Lengthen your body, with your head held high and your chin up. Aim your gaze about twenty feet in front of you rather than down toward your feet.
- Relax your shoulders and neck by rolling each shoulder forward, up, and back, then letting both shoulders drop down, gently pinching the shoulder blades together.
- Bend your elbows and allow your arms to swing freely, keeping them close to your body. You will naturally fall into a rhythm, bringing the opposite arm and leg forward together.
- Take short strides, striking the heel first, and then pushing off with your toes. Use your buttock muscles to propel you forward with each step.

Incorporate more walking into your day:

- Go down the hall to speak with a coworker instead of using the phone or email.

- Take the stairs rather than an elevator.
- Give up that close parking spot.
- Take a ten-minute stroll after meals.

If you are motivated by goals or data, get a pedometer. Aim for two thousand steps per day at first, then gradually work up to ten thousand. And remember that you don't have to do it all at once. It's the amount over the course of the day that counts.

Find a walking buddy. Getting support from others and enjoying what you are doing are both big contributors to success. Walking and talking with a friend or a beloved pet will help ensure that you stay with it.

Nonexercise Is the New Movement

We recently heard of a teen whose therapist insisted that he add exercise to help treat his depression. He hated the thought of exercise, so he came up with his own creative solution: "I'll put on my headphones, play loud music, and dance like crazy." That works!

Researchers at the Mayo Clinic have a fancy term for it: "Nonexercise Activity Thermogenesis" (NEAT). NEAT is any movement that is not done for the sake of fitness. *Thermogenesis* has to do with metabolism: it means that you burn calories with movement of any kind, even things like pacing the floor, tapping your toes, or chewing gum.[26]

Here are some additional ideas for healthy nonexercise movements. We've added the metabolic equivalent (MET) figures just for your interest. MET is a way of measuring the energy expended by various activities. Sitting and watching TV is rated at a MET level of 1.0. We'll use that as the number to beat.

- strolling (2–3 METs)
- cooking (2–3 METs)

- housecleaning (3–4 METs)
- fishing (3–4 METs)
- leisure biking (3–6 METs)
- lawn mowing/yard work (4–6 METs)
- gardening (4–6 METs)
- dancing (5–7 METs)
- hiking (6–8 METs)
- sexual activity (1.3–2.8 METs)

(Source: Compendium of Physical Activities[27])

You get the picture. Any movement above and beyond sitting and watching TV burns calories, raises your metabolism, and does good things for your brain. Move any way you like. Just move.

The Second Movement: Adagio

Adagio literally means "at ease" and describes music performed at a slow and stately pace. We call this "mindful movement," which to us means slow, flowing, graceful movement done with purposeful awareness. Whether you consider yourself to be graceful or not makes no difference. It is the quality of being present that matters.

Any movement that you do, you can do with greater awareness and presence. You can incorporate mindfulness into any of the above activities or into the more vigorous movements that follow. Still, there are tried-and-true types of movement, tested over the centuries, that build mindfulness into the very practice itself. We will focus on two of these: yoga and tai chi.

Yoga: Grace, Strength, and Balance

Yoga offers so many benefits that we believe a complete movement program could consist of just two things: walking and yoga. Yoga is peaceful and calming yet can be vigorous at times. It involves gentle stretching but also resistance (strength) training. It is especially good for the core muscles that are so important for maintaining posture, and it is great for people with back pain. And yoga can be done, with slight modifications, at any age.

Jean Fraser, owner of Soma Ventures, is a dancer turned yoga teacher. She created the yoga component for our Pathways to Resilience programs. We find these sequences to be especially helpful because they are designed to balance what we call the three mind states. These are the common but unpleasant mental states that we all fall into from time to time: anxious mind, agitated mind, and sluggish mind.

Yoga and breath practices help us to cultivate particular feeling states and qualities of mind. When anxiety is present, we can cultivate stability and calm. When we're feeling agitated, we can disperse that agitation through movement and breath. When we're feeling such low energy that the thought of accomplishing the simplest task is over-whelming, we can employ these simple movements to lure ourselves toward vitality and alertness. These practices engage the body to help the mind. Choose any one of these to add some movement when you stand up throughout the day. Or do them all in sequence to change the state of your mind. If you would like to purchase a video to guide your practice, refer to the Resources section at the back of the book.

Tai Chi: Breath, Movement, and Awareness

Tai chi (or its meditative partner qigong) is another great option for mindful movement. It is slow, gentle, and flowing—and can raise and sustain energy without being overly stimulating. It is a perfect addition to movement as we age, in part because it incorporates balance and memory. Learning the new postures and sequences, much like learning a new dance, helps stimulate the production of new neural pathways. And because it is so calming to move and breathe in this way, it can help tone down the stress response, further protecting our brains.

It is beyond the scope of this chapter to describe how to do this elegant practice. We would encourage you to find a good teacher or a video to guide you. Our colleague, Marie Overfors at Evergreen Fitness in Minneapolis, has developed a teaching video that is easy to learn and perform at any age. The gentle, flowing movements of this particular type of tai chi are especially good for keeping our bodies (and our minds) supple, strong, and flexible as we age. Please refer to the Resources section for information on how to order this video.

The Third Movement: Allegro

Allegro movements are fast, quick, and bright. This is *active movement*, usually referred to as "exercise." It can be as vigorous and intense as you'd like it to be, so long as you approach it safely, with the caveats listed above (see the Physical Activity Readiness Questionnaire). If you have any questions about your own readiness, or if you have been physically inactive for some time, this would be the time to consult with your doctor.

Aerobic exercise gets most of the attention in this arena, but we're going to emphasize two other types of active movement that we think offer the most benefit for brain health: interval training and progressive resistance.

Staccato Movements: Get the Most Out of Movement with Bursts of Activity

Let's revisit the fight-or-flight response and the good stress that can come from movement. The kind of movement that is called for when survival is really at stake involves brief, intense bursts of activity, followed by periods of recovery. We are wired for this. As children, we did active bursts all the time, because it was incorporated into play. But adults tend to avoid this type of movement, in part because it can be uncomfortably hard. Why would we want to work so hard if we don't have to?

One reason is that high-intensity interval training may be the most efficient, most effective, most beneficial to the brain of all forms of movement. Interval training does the following:

- promotes weight loss, especially for that hard-to-lose abdominal weight.[28]
- raises your metabolic rate for twenty-four to forty-eight hours, burning calories long after you've stopped exercising.[29]
- improves levels of hormones including cortisol, testosterone, and human growth hormone.[30]
- protects against adult-onset diabetes.[31]
- boosts energy, focus, and performance.
- helps slow the aging process.

All these benefits contrast favorably to low-intensity aerobic exercise, which most of us have thought is the way to go if we want to get healthier and lose weight. In fact, new research suggests that slow endurance exercise may actually *promote* the storage of fat by raising cortisol levels.[32] We're not suggesting that you drop your long, slow movement routines, because we believe they have many other advantages. But you ought to consider adding occasional brief, intense bursts of movement to your weekly routine.

Below is an interval training plan that you can adapt to whatever activity you prefer. Choose an activity you like that can be done intensely in brief spurts (twenty to thirty seconds is enough). Good options include walking or running, biking, rowing, using a treadmill or elliptical trainer, swimming, calisthenics, or dancing. Get creative.

Before you start, remember to run your plan by your doctor, especially if you have not been active in some time. Then start slowly. You can build the intensity as you become more fit. When you're first starting out, just make the bursts a little faster and harder than your usual pace. Do the program once or twice a week. You will get all the good effects you need from just two sessions of ten to fifteen minutes per week.

Interval Training Program

Begin with 2–3 minutes of warm-up, doing your chosen movement at a comfortable pace.

Then go faster and harder for 20–30 seconds. If you're just starting out, simply pick up the pace a bit. As you progress, you can gradually push yourself harder until you go as fast as you possibly can, but just for 20–30 seconds. That's all you need.

Slow down to a recovery pace, similar to your warm-up pace. Give yourself 1–2 minutes for recovery.

Repeat with another 20–30 second burst of activity, followed by 1–2 minutes of recovery. Do this for 3–4 cycles at first, gradually working up to 6–8 burst/recovery cycles.

This entire workout takes only ten to fifteen minutes, but the effects will last for days. Do this once or twice per week and you will boost your metabolism, sharpen your mind, and slow the aging process.

Keep Yourself Strong

Want to create stronger bones, protect your joints, improve your sleep, tone your body, improve your mood, prevent falls, *and* promote growth of new brain cells? Then add one or two sessions of progressive resistance movement per week.

Progressive resistance simply means that you get stronger by adding more resistance over time. You can do this in several ways: yoga, resistance bands, weight machines, free weights, or using the weight of your own body. Even some gardening chores count as resistance training if they involve things like lifting, digging, or hauling.

Our colleague Dave Wieber is a gifted physical therapist who knows a lot about how to keep the body strong and resilient as we move from youth to middle age and beyond. He has helped thousands of people recover their movement after injury—even helping to keep Dr. Emmons active for the past twenty years! His work as both a physical therapist and a trainer have taught him to value functional movement and core strength over the beach-body physique that we may have wanted when we were younger.

Dave has designed a total body resistance workout that includes all the major muscle groups. It is progressive, with three levels of difficulty, and it requires no expensive equipment because it uses your own body weight to provide the resistance. Best of all, there is almost no risk of injury; in fact, his program is designed to *prevent* injury as we age. If you want a great workout that you can do in your own home, you may want to purchase his video, *Fit after 40*. (See *Resources* in the appendix.)

Before starting your program, refer to the Physical Activity Readiness Questionnaire above. If you are new to resistance training, we recommend that you consult with a trainer, who can help you choose the best exercises and show you proper technique to avoid injury.

Progressive Resistance Training Program

Start slowly, with a low amount of resistance and increase the resistance gradually.

Include all the major muscle groups: legs, hips, back, chest, abdomen, shoulders, and arms. Use enough resistance that it is hard to do more than 8–12 repetitions without assistance. One set for each exercise is enough.

- If you want greater intensity or to build your strength more quickly, make the movements slower. Count to ten as you move the weights away from you, and again as you bring them back down. Use as much weight as you can lift for only 3–6 repetitions.
- If you do a total body resistance workout using your own body weight, as in the *Fit after 40* program, you can do it up to three times per week.
- If you use free weights or weight machines with 8–12 reps, then twice a week is sufficient.
- If you do the slow movement with maximal weights (3–6 reps), limit it to once per week.

The Coda: Movement for a Lifetime

Now let's put it all together and show you how to craft your own life-long movement plan. But first, a few words of advice:

Movement should be fun. It ought to be something you want to do. The best way to ensure that you will move is to keep it fresh, to do many different things that you enjoy. Keep it light and playful. Move with others whenever you can. Most important, just move.

◇◇

A Helpful Practice

The Best-Laid Plans: An "Ideal" Movement Plan

The following offers a perfect way to move your body—not too little, not too much—and incorporates all the forms of movement (and rest) that your body craves.

Every Day

- Stand up every 15–20 minutes throughout the day. Never sit for extended periods without moving against gravity.
- Incorporate a variety of nonexercise movements throughout each day.
- Walk for 30–45 minutes several days during the week. Or bike, ski, row, or whatever movement you prefer, at a light to moderate pace.

Twice a Week

- Do 10–15 minutes of high-intensity interval training.
- On alternate days, do some form of medium weight-bearing/resistance work (such as yoga, gardening, a total body resistance workout, or light weight lifting).
- Add a mind-body movement like yoga or qigong. Go to a class or use a home video to guide you.

Once a Week

- Do a slow resistance circuit (weight training) using maximal weights with minimal repetitions (3–6).
- Take a day of rest.

◇◇◇

Let's Get Real: The Good-Enough Plan

Not able to live up to the ideal? No worries, the plan that follows will still get you what you want—a more youthful, vibrant brain.

- Stand up as often as you can. Try to remember not to sit for too long without moving.
- Walk (or do another light aerobic activity) more days than

not. Pick up the pace a few times, for just a minute or so, then slow it down again.

- Do some sort of weight-bearing activity at least once a week.
- Try to get 20 minutes of focused activity most days of the week. Just 20 minutes early in the day will give you most of the benefit from movement, and the effects will last the whole day.

If You Do Just One Thing

We offer here a way to combine nearly all of what we have recommended into one simple activity—*mindful walking with nasal breathing*. You can set aside twenty minutes for this, or just make it part of your regular daily activities. Try not to see it as "exercise" or even as a means of getting from one place to another. Just walk for the pleasure of walking.

- If possible, go outdoors, preferably in a natural setting.
- Try to notice as much as you can about your experience: the movement of your body, your breathing, and all of your senses.
- Vary your pace, noticing how different it feels to stroll leisurely or to quicken to a more vigorous pace.
- Try breathing deeply in and out through your nose. Keep doing this as you vary your pace, and see if you can keep the breath long and slow, through the nose, even as you move more quickly.
- Remember, you have nowhere to go, and nothing to do but to be fully where you are. You are simply enjoying movement for its own sake.

5

A Youthful Brain Is Well Rested

Key 2

Young ones, don't waste your courage
racing so fast,
flying so high.

See how all things are at rest—
darkness and morning light,
blossom and book.

—RAINER MARIA RILKE

Key Concepts

- Rest, especially sleep, is the most nonnegotiable lifestyle measure for good brain health. Yet most of us are chronically sleep-deprived.
- While we continue to need about the same amount of sleep as we age, sleep patterns do change. Sleep *problems*, however, are preventable.
- Sleeping well is the most powerful means we have to promote mood, memory, and healing.
- There are two physiological events occurring during healthy sleep that seem to make it such a magic elixir: it regulates our internal clock, and it cleans out the brain.

Life is inevitably stressful, and taming the stress monster is so important that much of this book addresses it in one way or another. In the previous chapter we discussed how movement helps dissipate the stress response, and the next chapter will look at the role of diet. Later chapters will look closer at the mind-body connection so that you can use the power of your own mind to keep yourself well.

The focus of this chapter is on rest, and particularly on sleep. This is such a simple source of resilience that it is often overlooked, yet sleep may be *the* essential key to brain health. Sadly, not many of us are getting the kind of rest we need to sustain a youthful brain.

Sleep: The National Deficit

We are a sleep-deprived nation. According to the Centers for Disease Control and Prevention, insufficient sleep is a public health epidemic, and it is mostly one of our own making. Sleep experts agree that most adults need seven to eight hours of sleep per night, yet one third of working adults fall far short. The average adult sleeps closer to six hours per night, whereas just a few generations ago most people enjoyed an average of nine hours of sleep per night. Because we are so sleep-deprived, nearly 50 percent of people of all ages now report unintentionally falling asleep during the daytime. A frightening number admit to doing so while driving![1]

While lack of sleep is often by choice or poor sleep habits, many people simply *can't* sleep well. Insomnia affects as many as 85 percent of adults in any given year. Chronic insomnia—difficulty sleeping for a month or more—affects 10 to 15 percent of US adults at any given time.[2] Sleep disturbances are more common among women than men, and they become more frequent with age.[3] The economic costs are staggering: a recent estimate put the direct costs from insomnia at $14 billion annually in the United States alone.[4] The indirect costs are far higher.

What Happens to Sleep As You Age

Many people believe that the older we get, the less sleep we need. According to the National Sleep Foundation, sleep patterns do indeed change and more people are dissatisfied with their sleep as they age. But it is not true that we *need* less sleep, just that we *get* less quality sleep.

For sleep to be effective, the brain needs to cycle through periods of lighter and deeper sleep several times per night and also to experience the active dreaming that occurs during REM sleep. With age, many people spend more time in the lighter sleep stages, awaken more easily, and spend less time in the deep or dreaming phases of sleep.[5] These changes, which have dramatic health consequences, are caused by many factors, including

- illnesses and the medications used to treat them
- changes in circadian rhythm (our inner twenty-four-hour clock)
- hormone changes in women experiencing menopause
- prostate problems in men
- gut issues like indigestion or heartburn
- an increased proportion of belly fat that heightens both gut and hormone problems
- lowered melatonin production in the brain
- increased levels of cortisol

While we can all expect some changes in sleep patterns over the years, we intend to show you that sleep *problems* like those above are not inevitable as we age. The science of sleep is progressing rapidly, and there is already much knowledge that we can apply to sleep better. We will share with you what we consider to be the best information and most effective strategies to get yourself resting better and feeling younger, no matter what your quality of sleep has been until now.

What Rest Does for Your Brain

For the last half century or so, sleep researchers have been trying to understand *why* we sleep. What is so important about sleep that we spend roughly one third of our lives in slumber, seemingly not accomplishing anything productive? Why has sleep persisted in every species throughout all of evolution, even when the act of sleeping leaves one so unprotected?

Until recently, it has been assumed that there must be a single unifying benefit to sleep that no one has yet been able to discover. Now we're realizing that there isn't just one thing, but many crucial ways that sleep helps both body and mind. Here we will focus on three of the most important: mood, memory, and healing.

Sleep Improves Your Mood

"I was working really hard on a project, so I went for a couple of nights without much sleep. The next day my mood was up. I felt great! But then I crashed and got so depressed I had to be taken to the hospital."

Karla had a mood disorder for which she had just begun treatment. But when she chose to shortchange her sleep in order to work on her project, she unwittingly triggered severe mood swings, first up and then very down. One of the primary benefits of sleep, more powerful than most of us realize, is to keep our moods brighter and more stable.

It has long been known that there is a connection between problems with sleep and depression. Until recently, it has been assumed that insomnia is a *symptom* of depression, and it will improve when the depression is treated. But research is now showing that it goes in the other direction as well. Poor sleep, as Karla found out, is one of the most common *causes* of depression. In fact, it appears that chronic insomnia (trouble sleeping for a month or more) doubles one's risk of developing depression.[6]

On the flip side, a recent study found that reducing insomnia doubles the chances of recovering from depression. The researchers did not use sleeping medications or antidepressants to treat insomnia. They used cognitive behavioral therapy for insomnia (CBT-I), a brief talk therapy that teaches people to develop good sleep patterns and learn to tame their minds. Most people who receive this therapy greatly improve their sleep, and when they do, they have an 87 percent chance that their moods will return to normal. In those who continue to sleep poorly, only half as many recover from depression.[7]

One of the means by which sleep improves mood is that it reduces what is known as *emotional reactivity*. You may recall the amygdala, located in the brain's emotional center, which sets off the alarm bells when we feel threatened or frightened. If it is overreactive, the amygdala is a bit like a young child who lacks the ability to soothe himself when upset. The child needs a calm, steady parent to help settle him down.

Most of us as adults have a well-functioning prefrontal cortex (the PFC) that acts like that good parent and soothes our emotions when we are upset. Just like real parents, however, the PFC remains calm and effective more easily when we've slept well. As Dr. Matthew Walker, a sleep scientist at the University of California, Berkeley, explains, "In people who've had a good night of sleep, the connection between the deep brain and the prefrontal cortex has been refreshed or restored. As a consequence, the frontal lobe is able to regulate—in a socially appropriate, psychologically controlled way—the emotional amygdala."[8]

Sleeping poorly, even for one night, is like changing the sensitivity on a dial, making you feel everything more intensely. A good night's sleep, on the other hand, helps dial it back down so that you react much less strongly to things, even if you face the exact same challenges the following day. This ability to withstand life's stresses and still maintain a healthy mood is known as emotional resilience, or *stress hardiness*. It goes a long way toward preventing psychological conditions like anxiety and depression. It may also protect against degenerative disorders like dementia.

There is a strong correlation between emotional resilience and quality of sleep. For example, researchers recently looked at a similar trait they called *mental toughness*, "the display of confidence, commitment, challenge, and control" among adolescents.[9] They found that teens with high mental toughness slept more deeply and efficiently, with fewer awakenings, less light sleep, and less daytime sleepiness. They also proved to be more resilient and better adjusted throughout adolescence and into adulthood. It is believed that mental toughness reduces stress levels, allowing for better sleep, but it likely goes in the other direction as well: better sleep enhances mental toughness.

Good sleep also takes the edge off emotionally painful events. When you dream, there is a dramatic drop in a stress chemical called norepinephrine (the brain's equivalent to adrenaline). This means that you are in a much less stressed state during REM sleep, even if you're dreaming about stressful events. Researchers think that this may allow you to work through painful memories in a stress-free state.[10] It's as if you are giving yourself free therapy as you sleep!

Sleep Clears Your Mind

"I'm really concerned about my memory. Some days it's fine, but there are more and more times at work when I just don't seem to function well. I'm afraid that someday I'm going to make a big mistake and lose my job because of it."

Robert was in his late fifties, an age when memory concerns often crop up. He feared that he was showing signs of dementia, but when he began to track his focus and memory, he realized how much they were affected by his sleep. Whenever he had a good night's sleep, his mind worked so much better that he felt twenty years younger. His experience illustrates a second great benefit of rest—it clears the mind and helps with focus, concentration, and memory.

A recent study at Berkeley confirmed the link between memory loss and poor sleep. They found that brain waves occurring during deep sleep transfer memories from the hippocampus to the cortex, where they are then stored long-term. But sleeping poorly impairs this process so that the memories cannot be transferred, effectively becoming *stuck* in the hippocampus.[11] This becomes a greater issue with age, because the older we get, the less time we spend in deep sleep. That in turn results in forgetfulness, like the inability to remember names or numbers, which was causing Robert such concern.

Researchers think that there are three important ways that deep sleep impacts learning and memory. When you sleep deeply *before* learning something new, it sets you up to move that new information efficiently from short-term to long-term storage. Secondly, sleeping well *after* learning helps by cementing those new memories into the long-term storage area. The third impact has more to do with creativity: during deep sleep your brain makes connections between seemingly unrelated threads, helping you to see their commonalities and relationships.[12] This may be why you can wake up with a new insight or a solution to a problem that was vexing you just the day before, and it shows the wisdom of the suggestion "Let's sleep on it."

Sleep Repairs Your Body

"I am tired all the time, no matter how much I sleep. I want to exercise, but I just can't. Some days, I can barely move. I've gained so much weight and my whole body hurts—all my muscles feel tender and sore. It never lets up!"

Joanne has been under such stress for so long that she never sleeps well anymore, leaving her body unable to repair and restore itself in the deeper stages of sleep. After years of this pattern she was left with constant pain and fatigue, as well as weight gain that she couldn't shake in spite of her constant dieting.

The underlying cause for Joanne's suffering is the same problem that now affects a high percentage of adults: systemic inflammation (inflammation affecting the whole body). We will return to this topic in the next chapter, because diet has so much to do with it. But even if your diet is healthy, the flames of inflammation can be fanned by inadequate sleep.

A very large and long-term study, known as the Heart and Soul Study, recently looked at the impact of sleep quality on systemic inflammation. Over a five-year time span, researchers measured several biomarkers (C-reactive protein, interleukin-6, and fibrinogen) associated with inflammation. Their interest was in heart disease, but inflammation affecting the heart will also affect the brain. They found that poor-quality sleep was in fact associated with greater inflammation and higher risk of heart disease. But there were differences based upon gender. Women who slept less than six hours per night were two and a half times more likely to have elevated markers of inflammation, especially if they awakened too early. Men, however, had less inflammation even if they slept poorly. These findings suggest that higher testosterone levels may protect men to some degree, whereas lower estrogen levels (for example, after menopause) may put women at greater risk from inflammation.[13] That's all the more reason to attend carefully to sleep *and* diet in the menopausal years.

Insufficient sleep can make it hard for people like Joanne to lose weight despite regular dieting. Poor-quality sleep leads to changes in the appetite-regulating hormones (ghrelin and leptin), which in turn can lead to overeating. Also, when healthy volunteers were sleep-deprived for just four nights, their fat cells were found to be insulin-resistant. This suggests that sleep may regulate energy metabolism throughout the body, and insufficient sleep may cause both obesity and prediabetes, leading to all kinds of health risks.[14]

A phone survey of nearly half a million people in all fifty states has confirmed the strong link between insufficient sleep and chronic health problems. They have found common conditions like high blood pressure, asthma, and arthritis are all associated with inadequate sleep, as are obesity, heart disease, and stroke. While this study is ongoing, the researchers are already concluding that lack of sleep plays a major role in most chronic diseases and should be addressed as part of an overall treatment program.[15]

Why Rest Works:
Of Brain Clocks and House Cleaning

How can sleep, which we take so for granted, have such a dramatic impact on our bodies and minds? To understand the magic of sleep, we need to look a little deeper into the molecular machinery of the brain. We will focus on two groundbreaking findings from recent neuroscience: chronobiology and the glymphatic system. Translated, these refer to our brain's biological clock and nighttime housekeeping.

The Importance of Aligning with Nature's Rhythms

You may not know it, but you have a clock in your brain. More accurately, most of the cells in your body have their own clock, and those clocks are all controlled by the brain's master timekeeper, called the *suprachiasmatic nucleus* (the SCN).

Within the cells throughout your body is an oscillating mechanism that serves as a timer, controlling everything from the cell's metabolism to your ability to respond to the day's varying demands. This timer is tied to our twenty-four-hour circadian cycle. Even the brain chemicals like serotonin and dopamine are closely linked to this biological rhythm. This system is orchestrated by the SCN, which is located in the hypothalamus deep within the brain. The SCN acts like a conductor, keeping all the other cells aligned in a complex rhythmic dance.

The SCN takes its cues from light, most notably the alternating day and night cycles known as circadian rhythms. Some people are genetically prone to being out of sync with nature's rhythms (for example, "night owls"), but everyone is susceptible to circadian disruptions, especially in today's world. The SCN is easily thrown out of alignment by various aspects of modern life such as electric lights, life stresses, and social norms (spend a night on a college campus to get an example of this last one).

Light exposure, the most important factor in keeping us biologically aligned, has changed dramatically in just a few generations. Merely a hundred years ago, most people spent a good deal of their day outdoors exposed to the bright light of the sun. In the evenings, lights were very dim (if there was any light at all). As a result, our ancestors would naturally become very sleepy within a couple of hours after sunset. If you have ever gone camping in a really dark place, you have probably experienced this for yourself. But since most of our time is now spent indoors, we risk getting too little light during the daytime and more light than we should at night.

Being out of alignment with circadian rhythms can quickly alter our physiology, triggering many of the health concerns described above. Just one night of sleep deprivation can impair learning and memory, reduce the function of the immune system, or unleash a psychiatric illness. Up to 90 percent of people with major depression have circadian-related sleep disruption, and there are even links between disruption of the biological clock and drug and alcohol abuse.[16]

Scientists have recently discovered a likely reason for this relationship between circadian rhythm disruption and illness. There are many genes that are regulated by our biological clock, particularly those genes associated with mood.[17] This may explain why there is such a strong link between the timing of sleep and our overall state of health and emotional well-being. Among the genes affected by insufficient sleep are those associated with metabolism, inflammation, the immune system, and the stress response. These changes in gene expression have been shown to occur within just *one week* of insufficient sleep in healthy volunteers.[18]

The connection between light exposure and mood is becoming so clear that it ought to change how we think about depression. For example, researchers looked at a large number of elderly people (516 individuals with an average age of 72.8) and their degree of exposure to light at night. They found a very strong correlation between depression and the amount of light in their bedrooms at night, and concluded that an important way to prevent depression may be to simply keep the bedroom light very low.[19]

Likewise, using bright light exposure early in the day is looking more and more like an effective treatment for depression, even if the depression has nothing to do with the time of year (as in seasonal affective disorder). One study done with elderly patients with nonseasonal depression found that an hour of bright light exposure in the morning for just three weeks lifted their moods and toned down their stress hormones, and the improvements continued even after the treatment was stopped.[20] It is also worth noting that light therapy, when it is properly used, may lift the mood faster and more strongly than antidepressants, and may work even if the depression has become chronic (lasting more than two years) and unresponsive to medications.[21]

Light exposure works via the brain chemical *melatonin*. Melatonin tells you what time your body thinks it is, regardless of what the clock says. When you are exposed to light before bedtime, for example, your body may misinterpret that signal, thinking that it is much earlier in the evening. This changes the timing and amount of melatonin released and has profound effects on sleep.

In 2011, researchers compared exposure to typical room light (200 lux) versus dim light (up to 3 lux) in the late evening with 116 healthy volunteers. In nearly *everyone* (99 percent), the room lights suppressed their secretion of melatonin, pushing back the timing of sleep and shortening the effects of melatonin by an average of ninety minutes. They also found that being exposed to room lights during sleep hours, even briefly, suppressed melatonin by 50 percent, leaving the body confused and acting like the night is much shorter than it is.[22] This may explain why so many people find themselves unable to get to sleep early enough even during the long nights of winter, a time when our bodies are craving more rest. This may also be one reason why it may be harder to fall back to sleep if you turn on the lights when you wake in the middle of the night.

We would do well to remember that our bodies have evolved to have an elegant relationship with the natural world. One of the most important and enduring aspects of this relationship is that we are tied to nature's rhythms, including the seasons, the months, and shorter cycles of activity and rest. The most powerful of these rhythms is the twenty-four-hour cycle that we call a day. If we stop to think about it, it makes complete sense to wake with the light, to wind down after dark, to be active when most of the natural world is active, and to sleep when it is time to sleep. We were designed to sleep deeply and to sleep long for good reason.

Sleep: The Great Detoxifier

You may be familiar with the lymphatic system, the body's means of waste management. Lymphatic vessels run parallel to the blood vessels, draining the metabolic waste products from all over the body toward the heart for eventual elimination. The system's jobs include clearing the body of potentially harmful byproducts of metabolism, as well as managing inflammation and immunity. But lymph does not clear the brain of its toxins, because the blood-brain barrier maintains the brain as a closed system.

Now a study just published in *Science* and considered one of the greatest scientific breakthroughs of the year, reveals how the brain does its housekeeping. It has its own system of channels, labeled the *glymphatic system*, which run parallel to the brain's blood vessels and clear out its waste products for eventual removal by the liver. But it does its work mainly at night, while we are asleep.

It may seem hard to believe, but brain cells appear to shrink by up to 60 percent during sleep in order to open up space for these glymphatic channels to flow. This system ramps up to become ten times more active while we are asleep than when we are awake. All this cleaning activity may explain why the brain uses nearly as much energy at night as it does during the daytime.[23]

One of sleep's primary purposes, then, may be to shut down the brain's usual activity so that the cleanup can begin. This is a bit like a busy office building that is filled with people and activity during the day. When it closes down for the night, other workers can come in to clean and prepare for the next day's work.

Likewise, it appears as if our brains have to choose between being active and alert, as during the daytime, *or* cleaning up, as happens at night. One of the study's authors, Dr. Maiken Nedergaard, explains that it's "like having a house party. You can either entertain the guests or clean up the house, but you can't really do both at the same time."[24]

This discovery has obvious implications for brain diseases like Alzheimer's, which is associated with the buildup of a protein called beta-amyloid, a waste product that should theoretically be cleared by this glymphatic system. There are many unanswered questions, of course, but this study certainly reminds us that, if we care about the health of our brain, we will not short ourselves of the precious and still-mysterious thing we call sleep.

How to Sleep Well

If it were easy, we'd all be sleeping soundly and naturally, night in and night out. But there are many things working against getting a good night's sleep, some that are self-imposed and others seemingly beyond our control. We want to bring some clarity and simplicity to the many recommendations that exist for improving sleep.

We will organize our suggestions into several layers. Some of you may only need to make a few simple adjustments; others will need to apply all the recommendations and keep working at them for a time. But we are confident that by following the system below, all of you can sleep better and experience the fruits of better rest: a happier mood, a clearer mind, a healthier body, and a more youthful brain.

Setting the Stage for Sleep, No. 1:
What to Do for Your Bedroom

The first and simplest step is to set up an environment that is conducive to sleep. For some, this may be all that you need to do, and all it takes are a few inexpensive details for your bedroom.

- Keep the bedroom for sleep. Remove work-related items, TVs, or other electronic devices. Keep the room simple and uncluttered.
- Keep it dark. Even small amounts of light can alter melatonin secretion, so shut out all possible lighting (including alarm clocks, cell phones, and night lights).
- Keep it quiet. When you cycle into a lighter stage of sleep, even the slightest sound can awaken you. If your partner snores, consider using a white noise machine (such as a room air cleaner). If need be, consider sleeping in separate rooms: studies show that most couples do sleep better in separate bedrooms.
- Keep it cool. You sleep best when your body is cooling, so keeping your room between sixty and seventy degrees is considered optimal.

- Keep it comfortable. Good bedding is obviously a plus for sleep, but it doesn't have to be expensive. The key may be to spend some time trying out a new mattress before you buy it. Consumer Reports says that spending fifteen minutes testing the bed in the store is as good as taking it home for a longer trial.

Setting the Stage for Sleep, No. 2: What to Do during the Day

Giving some attention to what we do during the rest of the twenty-four hours can pay off with an easier, deeper sleep.

- Get up gently, but do get up. It is crucial to get up at the same time every day (or close to it), because it sets your circadian rhythm. Avoid harsh alarms if possible, but use them if you have to. It's even more helpful to awaken with the light, either the natural sunrise or a "dawn simulator" (see Resources).
- Make your bed. One poll found that making your bed each morning improves the chances for a good night's sleep by nearly 20 percent, maybe because it keeps you from using your bed for anything but sleep.
- Get bright light. Take advantage of circadian rhythms by getting some exposure to bright light, preferably within an hour or two of waking. That will help regulate your natural melatonin cycle, improving your chances of getting sleepy at the right time of night. Natural sunlight is ideal, but if that's not possible, you can use a bright light device (see Resources).
- Move early and move often. There is no question that exercise can improve sleep; just don't leave it for too late in the day. The good stress of exercise is best avoided within

three hours of bedtime, to keep your stress hormones down and your body cool.

- Hold the caffeine. It's fine to enjoy caffeine drinks so long as you're sleeping well, but since its effects can last for twelve hours or more, it's best to stop well before noon.

- Eat early and eat light. If possible, have your largest meal at midday, when your body is more geared toward digestion. Eat lighter at the evening meal, but eat enough that you don't have to snack right before bed. Also cut back on the protein (it tends to be stimulating) and eat more healthy carbs (like whole grains, beans, root vegetables). This helps stabilize your blood sugar, allowing tryptophan to enter the brain, where it can make the calming chemical serotonin.

- Take care with alcohol. Like caffeine, alcohol is fine in modest amounts (usually defined as one drink for women, two for men) so long as you have no problems sleeping. But while having a drink right before bed might make you sleepy, it can cause problems two to three hours later when it wears off. Better to enjoy your drink with dinner.

- Take a few breathing breaks during the day. Simply stop what you're doing for a moment and turn your attention to your breath. Close your eyes if you can, but it is not essential. You don't need to do anything special with your breath, just try to experience it as fully as you can. You may want to notice the rise and fall of your belly, which helps you to naturally breathe more deeply. See if you can keep your attention fully on just three breaths. Do this as often as you think of it over the day. It only takes a minute. If you have a bit longer time, you may practice the calming breath technique (see below). Awareness of breathing can coax your autonomic nervous system to stand down and turn off your stress response.

Calming Breath

The calming breath addresses anxiety and stress by emphasizing the exhalation. When we are in a relaxed state, the exhalation is easeful, long and full, and there is no sense of needing to rush on to the next breath. When we are anxious or agitated, our mood is reflected in our breathing, which becomes shallow and rapid. We can cultivate a state of calm by consciously lengthening our exhalation.

- Settle into a comfortable seated position or lie down.
- Close your eyes and bring your attention to your breath. Slowly breathe in through your nose, counting to three or four.
- Pause briefly. Then gently exhale as you count to five or six so that the exhalations become longer than your inhalations.
- Continue in this way, without any sense of work or strain. As you follow your exhalations to the end, you may begin to notice a slight pause that occurs at the end of the breath. This is the wisdom of your body reminding you that within each breath cycle resides a brief stillness. By lengthening your exhalation and strengthening your connection to this pause, you strengthen your ability to cultivate and maintain a quality of calm.

Setting the Stage for Sleep, No. 3:
What to Do in the Evening

You're getting sleepy . . . very, very sleepy. Or at least you ought to be. Here are some steps you can take in the final hours before bed to help ensure a blissful sleep.

- Shut it down. Stop work of any sort at least an hour or two before bed, preferably sooner. What to do instead?

Try doing what our ancestors did—read a book, do some journaling, listen to light music, or spend time in prayer or meditation.

- Keep it dim. Turn off your electronics at least an hour before bed, including the computer, iPad, and smartphone. *Never* watch TV in bed. Keep the room lights as low as you can, or use candles. Darkness before bed will do amazing things for your natural sleepiness.

- Warm up to cool down. Take a warm bath or shower an hour or more before bed so that your body is in the cooling-down phase at bedtime.

- Get milk. A warm glass of milk (dairy, almond, soy, or other) before bed may in fact be good for sleep. The tryptophan deepens your sleep, and the warmth may simply be comforting. Add a small amount of cinnamon, cardamom, or nutmeg for an even more soothing drink.

The Final Act: What to Do at Bedtime

Now comes the easy part. All you need to do is lie down, close your eyes, and fall asleep. Here's how you can make that as easy as it sounds.

- Keep it regular. Aim to get to bed at about the same time each night. This habit is much easier if you get up at the same time each day.

- Go to bed when you're sleepy—but not before. While you want your bedtime to become regular, you also want to associate being in bed with sleeping, not lying there restlessly *trying* to get to sleep.

- Keep a routine. Just as when we were children, our bodies love a bedtime routine. Drink warm milk, brush teeth, go to bathroom, get in bed, read short bedtime story, lights off. Create your own routine, make it pleasurable, and tuck yourself in properly.

- Sleep on your side. Sorry if you're a back or stomach sleeper, but research tells us that you breathe easier, and sleep better, on your side. And if you ate too much or too late, start out on your left side: it's slightly easier on your digestion.

What about Naps?

Naps are great, so long as you are sleeping well at night. People who take short naps appear to learn better and solve problems more creatively. Smart companies encourage naps for their employees. Google, for example, has napping pods available to its workers. Here's how you can make a nap work for you:

- Time it right. You don't want daytime sleep to affect your circadian rhythm and make it hard for you to fall asleep at night. So keep it between the hours of noon and three p.m., assuming your bedtime is ten or eleven p.m.
- Keep it short. Einstein famously napped while holding a spoon. When he fell asleep, it fell to the ground, waking him immediately. A nap doesn't need to be that short, but keep it to thirty minutes or less. Sleeping longer often makes people groggier and can make it much harder to fall asleep that night.

What to Do If You Can't Sleep Well

Sleep hygiene (as above) provides a good foundation for sleep, but it is not always enough. So what do you do if you take all the above measures but still can't sleep well?

- First, you may have to let some things go. If you have insomnia for any reason, it's best to stop using *any* caffeine or alcohol, at any time of day. (If you're a regular caffeine user, you will need to reduce it slowly.) And also give up the naps until your sleep returns to normal.

- Next, add more bright light during the day. If possible, get outside for thirty minutes or more during the brightest time of day (solar noon). If you can't do that, consider getting a light box with 10,000 lux, or a blue-light emitter (see Resources). If you also have seasonal depression, trick your brain into thinking that the days are longer by using the lights early (between six and eight a.m.) and late (between five and seven p.m.) in the day.

- Take even more measures to keep your home dim in the evening. Get room-darkening shades for your windows if needed, or if they are too expensive, consider using an eye mask at night. Avoid any blue-wavelength light (even computer screens and clock radios), get dimmer switches for your living areas, and use light-blocking software for your computer or iPad (for instance, you can download a free app called f.lux).

- Go to bed only if sleepy, and get out of bed if you lie awake for twenty minutes or more. Go to a dark room and read something that's not overly exciting, or write in your journal. You may find it helpful to write down any worries so that you can stop running them through your head.

- To avoid ruminating about the fact that you can't sleep, do something to disengage your mind. You could try doing some math in your head, like counting backward from three hundred by threes. You might also try the calming breath technique (see above).

- Two scents: inhaling essential oils like jasmine and laven-
  der may be as effective as medications for reducing anxiety
  and helping sleep. You can add one to your bath in the
  evening or use a diffuser for your bedroom or simply place
  a drop of oil on your pillow. It works quickly, so you could
  try this before turning to the other natural therapies below.

What If You *Still* Can't Sleep?

It is tempting at this point to turn to medication, and we wouldn't
blame you if you did. But you may not want to give in just yet. Research on sleeping medications suggests that they aren't as helpful as
most of us think, adding just a few minutes of sleep per night, while
often contributing to memory issues or other side effects. In any event,
we don't see them as a long-term solution for sleep problems except in
a few conditions.

The natural therapies below are also intended for short-term use,
just until you can reestablish your natural sleep patterns. If you are taking other medications or have any questions about adding any of these
natural remedies, you should first consult with your doctor.

Melatonin:

Remember that melatonin is the brain chemical that regulates the
SCN, the brain's master clock. Melatonin is produced in the darkness,
and even normal room lighting can affect it. So first try to manage
your light exposure, as described above. However, melatonin production does decrease with age, and if you need more help *falling* asleep,
a small amount of a melatonin supplement can be safe and effective.

- Start with a very low dose (as little as .25 or .5 mg can
  work) about an hour before bed. If you get a sublingual

product (it dissolves under the tongue), you can wait until fifteen minutes before bed.

- You may gradually increase the dose every three or four days if needed. The usual dosage is between 1 and 3 mg, and you should not exceed 6 mg per night.
- Melatonin is considered quite safe, but it may still have some side effects. If you feel sedated, disoriented, or depressed, discontinue it.

Amino acids:

These natural substances come from proteins, but when taken alone they can have a mild medicinal effect. Whereas melatonin works best if you have trouble *falling* asleep, these can also be good for *staying* asleep. The two that we consider most helpful are tryptophan and L-theanine.

Your brain uses tryptophan to make serotonin, which is calming and conducive to sleep. It is plentiful in the diet, most notably in turkey and dairy. Your warm milk at bedtime may give you a good dose of this, but you can also take tryptophan, or its close cousin 5-HTP, in pill form. The usual dose is 500–1000 mg of tryptophan, or 50–100 mg of 5 HTP, taken about an hour before bedtime. Do not add to an antidepressant unless you have discussed it with your doctor.

L-theanine, which works with another calming brain chemical called GABA, can be especially helpful with anxiety. You get this in your diet too, most notably in green tea, but it is much more potent when taken as a supplement. The usual dose is 100–300 mg. Take it an hour or so before bed.

Herbal remedies:

Medicinal herbs have a long and well-documented history of safety and benefit. Though the effects may be mild compared to prescription medications, they can be a helpful and safe addition to your overall sleep program. There are many to choose from, and you may find it best to get a product that combines several, including hops, chamomile, and lemon balm. The two we find most effective for sleep are passionflower and valerian.

Passionflower doesn't sound like something that would promote restful sleep, but it can be very calming, and especially good when worry and anxiety are at play. The usual dose is 400 to 700 mg of freeze-dried extract, or 15 to 30 drops of liquid extract taken thirty minutes to an hour before bed.

Valerian root, often called "nature's valium," is a mild sedative with antianxiety properties. The dose ranges from 500 to 1500 mg in pill form, or 15 to 30 drops of liquid extract. Take an hour or more before bedtime.

Other mind-body solutions:

There are good studies suggesting that doing yoga, tai chi, or acupuncture during the daytime may improve sleep quality at night. Also consider finding a therapist who does cognitive-behavioral therapy for insomnia (CBT-I). It has been shown to be far more effective and longer lasting than medications for insomnia.

◇◇◇

A Helpful Practice

We leave you with this self-directed exercise using self-hypnosis to improve your sleep. Hypnosis can be a great tool for reestablishing restorative sleep because it involves three of the main elements necessary to fall into sleep most easily: *focusing attention, becoming absorbed in an experience,* and *increasing the responsiveness to suggestions.*

You may find it helpful to be guided in this sort of practice until you learn to do it on your own. See the Resources section for available CDs.

- To begin, sit down in a chair and assume a comfortable position. (As you practice the exercise and become more responsive to its suggestions, you can do the exercise in your bed.)

- Allow your eyes to look slightly upward while focusing on something stationary in the room, even if the room is dark.

- While continuing to focus your attention in this way, take note of your breath cycle, counting each circuit of inhale as it transitions to exhale as one complete circuit of breath. Count twenty of these cycles in total, going first from one to ten and then counting down again from ten to one.

- By now you may notice subtle changes that have already begun to occur. Your eyelids may be fluttering closed more often and may even choose to remain closed. Your breathing rhythm may be deepening and slowing. Your muscle tension may be flowing out with each exhale. Simply and gently allow these changes to occur.

- Then, when you find your attention has softened, form an image in your mind's eye of a large home, a comfortable, warm, but very large home with many rooms, with your bedroom tucked away in a corner of the home. Visualize that each room is illuminated by a candle. Start at the room farthest from your imagined bedroom. Quietly go into that room. Approach the candle and look into the flame. Then, with your next exhale, gently blow out the candle, then return to the hallway where the light of other candles lights the way. Walk now to the next room and once again, gently blow out the next candle. Continue this way, moving silently from room to room, noticing the hush that spreads across the house as you turn out each light, as though you become more and more quiet and sleepy just as the blowing out of each candle makes the house darker and more peaceful.

- As you draw closer to your bedroom, with the house silent and at rest, you can feel the boundary between your external senses and your mind's imagination blurring, as you are gently sliding into sleep. As you reach your bedroom and draw back the sheets, you can feel the spreading sensation of your body's longing to rest, to lie down with your head sinking into your pillow, and to effortlessly drift further into deep, restful sleep. Just allow that to happen . . .

- You may well fall asleep in the chair. That is okay. The key is to help yourself recognize that since you can fall asleep in a chair, you can certainly fall asleep in your own bed. When you are ready to transfer this learning from chair to bed, go ahead, keeping aware that you can construct the sleeping house to be as large or small as you need it to be in your mind's eye, with just enough candlelit rooms to allow the day to fade and for the experience of restful sleep to be the gift that awaits you as you and your imagination return to bed for the night.

This exercise targets a problem that you have no doubt experienced—the tendency to lie awake ruminating about the fact that you are not sleeping. Often we think that not sleeping is a problem that can be solved through effort. It is not. There is nothing we have to do to get to sleep. The paradox of sleep is that you can't achieve it by trying. You have to allow yourself to fall into sleep. You have to let go. That's easier said than done, but by practicing this and the other suggestions in this chapter, we are confident that you will sleep easier.

6

A Youthful Brain Is Well Nourished

Key 3

Eat food. Not too much. Mostly plants.
—MICHAEL POLLAN

Key Concepts

- Diet has a vital impact on brain health, for good or for ill. The underlying cause of disease often lies in what we put into our mouths. So does the source of health.
- Science is homing in on how a well-nourished brain sets you up for vital aging.
- Do you need supplementation? This is currently a hot controversy, and we will try to sort it out and offer sound advice on whether, and how, to augment your diet with herbal and nutritional supplements.
- How should you eat to protect your brain as you age? We will offer a brain-supporting approach to diet that is rooted in science and practical to use.

It should be easy and natural to nourish our bodies and brains. Yet in spite of all that we know about nutrition, the average diet today is less healthy than in previous generations. Eating right has become incredibly confusing in the twenty-first century. If you pay attention to the numerous books, blogs, and programs about diet, the contradictory information can leave your head spinning.

This chapter is intended to cut through the confusion and to offer a simple, sustainable way to both nourish and protect your brain as you age. As in our previous chapters, we will sift through the scientific findings, call upon our own experience, and hopefully add some common sense to the discussion about how to eat well.

What's Wrong with the Modern Diet? Plenty.

Pollan's first imperative above is "Eat food." Why even bother to say that? Shouldn't that be obvious?

No, it's not obvious, because much of what we eat isn't food. Anything that has been changed from its natural form is no longer real food. Few of us are old enough to remember what was stocked in grocery stores before an entire industry grew up around processing and packaging the food that we eat. But in historical terms, it is a very recent phenomenon. Breakfast cereal may have been the first modern processed food, and that began in earnest less than a century ago. It started as a well-meaning way to get more whole grains into the diet, but a walk down any cereal aisle will quickly tell you what has happened since. The food industry has become expert at making food taste good (usually by adding sugars and fats), making it convenient, and, with the help of our government, making it inexpensive. Unfortunately, the food industry has seldom made things healthier.

Along with the shift toward processed foods, there are several trends in recent decades that have dramatically changed the nature, and the healthiness, of our diets:

We eat less fiber. Besides removing key nutrients, processing foods breaks them down so that they have less fiber and require less effort to digest. That can lead to spikes in blood sugar that wreak havoc on our metabolism.

Sugar consumption has skyrocketed. Speaking of metabolic havoc, the amount of sugar we consume has increased dramatically over the past thirty years. This corresponds to the rise of the cheap and ubiquitous sweetener *fructose* (as in high-fructose corn syrup), which shows up in the majority of soft drinks and processed foods. We know it's not good for us. Now a current JAMA study confirms that added sugar consumption is driving up mortality from heart disease, *doubling* the risk of heart-related deaths in high-sugar users.[1]

We have become completely confused about dietary fats. Years ago, those who tried to eat healthfully were told to give up the "bad" saturated fats found in meat, butter, and dairy in favor of margarine and other hydrogenated oils. Now we know that hydrogenated oils are unhealthy, while the whole notion of whether saturated fats are really so bad is being questioned. A large international study found no evidence that saturated fats cause heart disease, or that adding unsaturated fats will protect you against heart disease.[2] Findings like this may overturn decades of firmly held beliefs about nutrition. Dr. Frank Hu, a Harvard epidemiologist, stated in response to this study, "The single macronutrient approach is outdated. I think future dietary guidelines will put more and more emphasis on real food rather than giving an absolute upper limit or cutoff point for certain macronutrients."[3]

We no longer get enough omega-3 in our diets. Our ancestors ate a lot of wild game and grass-fed animals. Like fish, the meat from those animals was naturally high in omega-3 fats because their own diets contained a lot of omega-3. Since omega-3 helps shut down inflammation and improves neuron function, it is essential for brain health. The grains consumed today both by us and by our domestic animals have a much lower omega-3 content. And since we now cook mostly with oils rich in omega-6 (including corn, safflower, and soy), we have gone from an equal ratio (1:1) to a dramatic inequality (20:1) of omega-6 to omega-3. In practical terms, that means that we have less ability to turn off inflammation, one of the major factors in chronic illness.

We eat very different grains. Modern wheat, *the* staple in many people's diets today, is far different from the variety of wheat our grandparents ate. Today, wheat has become a monoculture (that is, one available strain of wheat today versus many in the past) and it is less nutritious than past varieties. But the biggest problem from a health standpoint may come from its proteins (gluten and lectin). Today's wheat contains more protein, and it creates stronger reactions in many people, further contributing to inflammation.

We eat more, period. Obesity levels have gone up dramatically since the 1970s. According to a recent Gallup poll, only about a third of Americans are now normal weight, with 35 percent overweight and another 27.2 percent classified as obese.[4] In just thirty years, the average American's calorie consumption went up a whopping 30 percent, even though fat consumption decreased.[5] The culprits? Most of those added calories come from refined grains and sugars: super-sized servings, sodas, and snacks.

Surely we can do better than this, and after reading the next section, you'll *want* to!

Why Eat Better?
The Scientific Foundation for a Vital Brain

No one needs to be convinced that eating well is good for your health. We've been hearing it for decades, and we all know from our own experience that we just feel better when we choose healthier foods. Yet the scientific findings keep coming, making an ever more compelling case that what we put into our mouths has a profound impact on how we think, feel, and act. It's important to remember too that while the effects from food are immediate, they are also lasting. What we eat today will influence the state of our brains and bodies months, even years from now. And as you'll see, what we put into our *own* bodies may impact the health of our children—and even *their* children!

You Can Protect Your Brain:
Reduce the Risks of Sugar, Stress, and Inflammation

As we've said before, losses of memory and brain volume are *not* normal aspects of aging. But the brain is a highly sensitive organ, vulnerable to damage if not protected. Three of the greatest threats to your brain come from excess glucose, metabolic stress, and inflammation. All three can be neutralized by diet.

One prominent theory of why we age focuses on a group of harmful compounds called *advanced glycemic end products*, or AGEs. They are implicated in many chronic diseases, such as diabetes and heart disease,[6] and they are increased by high blood sugar. They are also linked to Alzheimer's disease, where they are far more common than in normal brains. It is believed that they create the sticky clumps of protein, blood sugar, and brain cells that cause some neurons to function poorly and others to die prematurely.[7] Elevated blood sugar also heightens the damage caused to the blood vessels in the brain by the proteins found in Alzheimer's disease.[8]

Blood sugar appears to literally *shrink* the brain, and it may not take much to do it. Even if it measures in the high end of the normal range, blood sugar is associated with shrinkage of the hippocampus.[9] And the higher the blood sugar level, the worse it is for the brain. A study done by Group Health in Washington State found a striking correlation between elevated glucose and the onset of Alzheimer's: the higher the blood sugar, the greater the risk.[10]

Elevated blood sugar can, of course, be caused by a diet high in sugar or other simple (refined) carbs, like white breads, pastas, and corn products. But it is also caused by stress. The stress hormone cortisol tells you to eat. Not only that, but it tells you to eat the very things that quickly raise blood sugar—the refined sugars and grain products that we've just said put our brains at such risk.

Chronic stress is not just uncomfortable, it is harmful. Stress clearly impacts cognition and memory, and it increases your risk for Alzheimer's and other forms of dementia.[11] Problems with the stress response may partly explain why some people develop Alzheimer's while others can show the same microscopic changes associated with Alzheimer's in their brains and *not* get the disease. They must have some protective factor, but what? A recent discovery points to a protein that regulates the on-and-off switch for genes related to Alzheimer's— a protein that is part of the normal stress-response system.[12] There are built-in protections for the brain against the effects of aging. A healthy relationship with stress is one of them.

We will offer you effective strategies to reduce stress in later chapters. Meanwhile, don't underestimate the power of diet to protect you from it.

A different kind of stress, one that occurs at the cellular level, is known as *oxidative stress*. Your brain cells produce the energy they need through a process called *metabolic oxidation*. It is a complex and rather messy process, and there are toxic byproducts from oxidation that can be harmful to your brain. Fortunately, Mother Nature has provided for this side effect with protective elements in food. Foremost among them are a group of nutrients called *antioxidants*. As the name implies, they help to counter the harmful effects of oxidation and offer much-needed protection for the brain.

As we age, this metabolic process tends to get even messier, so we need that protection all the more. We will give more specific suggestions for brain-protective foods below, but the advice can be summarized simply: eat a large variety of brightly colored fruits and vegetables. The phytonutrients that give them their colors also give us the protection we need.[13]

A particularly unhealthy result of chronic stress is that it promotes inflammation. We should remember that inflammation, like the stress response, is a normal process. It is part of the body's protective system, warding off infections and promoting healing after injury. But like most states of activation, it is not meant to be on all the time.

Inflammation that affects the entire body is called *systemic inflammation*. Increasingly, it is linked to brain diseases, including dementia, strokes, and depression. Balancing blood sugar and insulin (the hormone that allows the cells to use glucose) can go a long way toward reducing inflammation. We'll give you the tools for balancing them later in this chapter.

You Can Improve Your Digestion: The Gut–Brain Connection

Another source of inflammation is the development of food sensitivities. We talked earlier about how dietary wheat has changed over the years, and you hear a lot these days about "gluten intolerance." Some of it is media hype, but it is also a real phenomenon.

Only a small percentage of people have full-blown celiac disease (an autoimmune disorder), but many more develop gluten intolerance. According to a Mayo Clinic study, this is not just an imagined problem, and it can carry serious health risks, many stemming from inflammation. They concluded that the higher rates of glucose intolerance are likely due to changes in eating habits (we eat more wheat products) and the more reactive form of wheat that we eat today.[14]

Here's how gluten sensitivity develops: Your immune system's job is to protect you from foreign invaders, and that includes food proteins like gluten. At first, you don't mind a little gluten. It's not really harmful unless you have celiac disease, so gluten is allowed to go through your digestive tract without complaint—for a while. But with repeated consumption of today's high-gluten wheat, the immune system eventually says "Enough!" and starts to react to it. When you develop inflammation in your intestines, it means that you have lost your tolerance to gluten, that is, you have become sensitive to it. That's when the real trouble begins.

Over time this intestinal inflammation can erode the integrity of the gut lining, a vital part of your body's defense system. Gut lining is like a specialized inner skin, highly selective about what it allows into the body, extracting what it needs and letting the rest move on through to be eliminated. Many of the things you eat are fine so long as they stay *within* the intestines, but they cause serious problems if they get into the bloodstream.

Inflammation of the gut lining allows for just such problems. In what is known as *leaky gut syndrome*, the weakened gut can allow gluten and other foreign proteins to cross the intestinal barrier and enter the bloodstream. That *really* annoys the immune system, which reacts with a fury, creating an inflammatory response that spreads systemwide. Unfortunately, the brain is especially vulnerable to this state of systemic inflammation.[15]

One reason this problem is increasingly common is that we eat so much wheat. Many who are health conscious have been told to consume grains daily, so they eat whole wheat or other gluten-filled grains (such as corn, rye, spelt, kamut) every single day. Our ancestors didn't do that because they *couldn't*. Wheat wasn't always available, so they'd have to turn to more seasonal foods. That resulted in their immune systems' getting a break from gluten, so they didn't become sensitive to it. One way out of this problem for us, then, is to not eat wheat so often.

There are other foods that can cause similar reactions. The most common are dairy, corn, eggs, and nightshade vegetables (tomatoes, eggplant, peppers). To find out if you have food sensitivities, or to go on a simple cleansing diet, see the Resources section for brain-supporting diet tools developed by integrative nutritionist Carolyn Denton.

There is another vital aspect of the digestive system that affects your brain more than anyone imagined until recently—the health of your gut bacteria. There is growing evidence that the microbes in your gut, known collectively as the *microbiome*, influence the function of your brain, your health, and your overall well-being.

One promising area of research involves the potential effect of probiotics on mood and anxiety. For example, when researchers replaced the gut microbes of anxious mice with that from fearless mice, their anxiety improved.[16] In humans, the health of adults' serotonin system (the soothing brain chemical that also regulates mood) seems to be influenced by the health of the microbiome during childhood.[17]

Someday soon there will be prescription medications containing specific probiotics to treat a range of diseases. Already, certain strains of gut bacteria have been shown to improve depressive behaviors in mice separated from their mothers, to reduce the stress response in humans,[18] and to give relief from anxiety, presumably by improving communication between the gut and the brain via the large nerve highway called the vagus nerve.[19]

We have been living with our own microbiome in a *symbiotic* (mutually helpful) relationship since birth, and our own health is dependent upon theirs. Microorganisms have been found to alter gene expression, immune function, body weight, and metabolism, and if the microbiome is healthy in childhood, adults have fewer autoimmune disorders, including type 1 diabetes, multiple sclerosis, rheumatoid arthritis, and even Alzheimer's disease.

The assault on the microbiome may explain why there's been an explosion of autoimmune and inflammatory disorders in the last fifty years. The hygiene hypothesis suggests that our obsession with germs and disinfection, plus our frequent exposure to antibiotics and other chemicals, is decimating our gut microbes, leaving us more susceptible to these illnesses.[20] "Our gut microbial community is an essential part of ourselves," explains Dr. Jayne Danska, a researcher in this area. "Bacterial cells outnumber human cells in our bodies by more than ten to one—and we live with them as partners."[21] We ought to treat them as such.

You Can Regulate Your Own Genes:
The Emerging Science of Epigenetics

"Food is information," says Carolyn Denton, an integrative nutritionist and our colleague at Partners in Resilience. In other words, what we eat is far more than just fuel to run our bodies. The nutrients in foods, both macronutrients (proteins, carbohydrates, and fats) and micronutrients (vitamins, minerals, probiotics), provide the information each cell needs to do its job.

Our DNA code, given to us at conception, provides a vital blueprint for the work of the cells. But DNA does not predetermine who we will become or what illnesses we will develop. It simply provides the code telling the cell what to do, for example what chemical enzymes to produce for its metabolism. DNA provides the blueprint, but whether or not various genes become manifest (known as *genetic expression*) depends upon many factors. One of the most important is the information the cell is given from food.

This means that what you eat plays a huge role in determining what illnesses you develop, whether that illness goes into remission, and whether it can be prevented in the first place. The science that studies how genetic expression develops is called *epigenetics*, and it is changing the way we think about health and disease. Scientists are finding more and more evidence that our lifestyle choices, such as our daily activities, the amount of stress we endure, and the food that we eat, influences which genes get expressed in our lives.[22]

There is emerging evidence that what we do with our own dietary choices may even influence generations to come. For example, one study found that if mice were overfed to the point of creating metabolic syndrome (obesity and insulin resistance), their offspring had this same tendency toward insulin resistance even if they did *not* overeat.[23] Something similar appears to happen in humans. Researchers in Sweden scoured historical records of crop yields and looked at health outcomes of future generations. They found that the *amount* of food available to fathers when they were young (just before puberty) correlated with their sons' likelihood of developing heart disease and their grandchildren's risk of diabetes. Scientists believe this occurs because epigenetic changes can get passed along to future generations, even though they are not actually part of the DNA code.[24]

In addition to heart disease and diabetes, there are two other age-related conditions that we know to be influenced by epigenetics: cancer and dementia. Many cancers, such as colon cancer, become far more common with both age and obesity. A process called *DNA methylation*, which determines whether genes are turned on or off, is strongly influenced by aging and overeating. But diet can also slow down methylation and reduce the risk of colon cancer. People with high vitamin D and selenium levels, for example, are at less risk of developing colon cancer.[25]

Memory-related diseases are also influenced by epigenetics, as was recently discovered by researchers in Spain. They found a specific gene that switches off as Alzheimer's disease advances, and since this gene regulates deposition of the tau protein (a pathological protein associated with frontotemporal dementia), it may be that the deactivation of this gene is one of the causes of dementia.[26]

Findings like these open up possibilities for new medications in the future, but they also give reason to hope that lifestyle measures that are known to influence these genetic switches (like diet and stress reduction) could even now help prevent conditions like Alzheimer's. Indeed, a thirty-five-year prospective study has already shown a 60 percent reduction in the risk of Alzheimer's disease (not to mention a 65 percent reduction in heart disease) in those who followed a healthy lifestyle—meaning regular exercise, a healthy diet, normal body weight, moderate alcohol use, and no smoking.[27]

Research by Dr. Dean Ornish and colleagues at UCSF suggests an even more remarkable idea: that aging may be *reversed* by the lifestyle choices we make! They followed men with low-risk prostate cancer for five years. Some were prescribed lifestyle changes (diet, activity, stress management, and social support), and others were not. The lifestyle change group actually lengthened their chromosome's *telomeres* (protective DNA at the ends of chromosomes) by 10 percent, while the control group lost about 3 percent of telomere length, a more typical change with aging.[28] Research out of Europe confirms that fruits and vegetables have a favorable effect on telomere length[29] and are associated with a greater lifespan.[30]

We choose to see this information as hopeful and we encourage you to do so too. *Your genes are not your destiny*. You can change them with the choices you make. Isn't it empowering to think that there is something you can do to influence the switching on and off of your genes? The food choices you make today will have a say in how healthy you are tomorrow, and next year, and into the coming decades. With all these reasons to eat better, let's learn how to do it.

Diet for a Youthful Brain

One of the fallacies of many diets is that they suggest that we should all eat the same way, that *this* particular diet is the right one for everybody. We don't see it that way. Each of us is different, and what's right for one person may not be for another. Some traditions, such as the ancient health system from India known as ayurveda (see *The Chemistry of Joy* for more details), honor those differences in their approach to diet, but many nutrition experts don't.

What we're offering here is not a diet per se, but rather an *approach* to diet. Many diets fail because they are too hard, too depriving, or too rigid, and most of us eventually rebel against such strict standards, even if we placed them upon ourselves. As Voltaire said, "The perfect is the enemy of the good."

We suggest that you start with the 51 percent solution: make the healthier choice more than half the time and you are still moving in the direction of better health. Over time, try to move that number up to 70 or 80 percent or more. Don't ever feel you have to follow these or any guidelines 100 percent of the time. Take a day off once in a while and enjoy eating whatever you want.

Should You Supplement?

Before we get to the guidelines, let's consider whether your diet is enough, or if you should consider supplementing it with nutritional products.

Half of all US adults take a daily vitamin, yet many doctors consider them to be worthless. A study just published in a prestigious medical journal seems to confirm their skepticism, leading a group of physicians to write an editorial in the same journal bluntly titled "Enough Is Enough: Stop Wasting Money on Vitamin and Mineral Supplements."[31]

The study, which followed male physicians sixty-five years and older, found that those who took a daily vitamin had the same amount of age-related cognitive decline as those who took a placebo pill. But the authors of the study cautioned that the study participants (all physicians) "may have been too well-nourished to observe benefits of supplementation." They added, "Further research is needed in other populations, such as those with nutrient deficiencies, to determine whether there are cognitive benefits specific to daily multivitamin use."[32] Critics of this study also point out that the vitamin they used (Centrum Silver) is a basic, low-dose vitamin that is not designed to have any impact on cognitive function.

Results published earlier *from the very same study* showed that a daily vitamin reduced risk of cancer and cataracts, and there are many other studies showing that supplements do have a positive effect on memory. For example, vitamin B12 and folic acid were shown to improve cognitive function in older men with depressive symptoms,[33] and B vitamins slowed the rate of brain atrophy in elderly subjects with early cognitive decline.[34] A very recent study found that an antioxidant supplement containing green tea and blueberry extracts, vitamin D, and amino acids improved the speed at which the brain processes information in older adults.[35] This is just a small sampling of positive findings resulting from natural therapies.

We believe it is best to meet your nutritional needs through diet, and the guidelines below will give you a good start on doing so. But we also think that there is a role for nutritional supplements, with plenty of research showing clear benefit when high-quality natural therapies are used intelligently under the right circumstances. While supplements will *not* compensate for repeated poor dietary choices, there are a few listed below with benefits that we believe are supported by the scientific research. Whenever it is feasible, we will include suggestions for how to get that nutrient in your diet.

Supplement	Why It's Important	How to Take It	Food Sources
B-complex vitamin (or a multivitamin with at least 500 mcg of B12, 20 mg of B6, and 800 mcg of folic acid)	B vitamins lower homocysteine, a harmful compound associated with inflammation and Alzheimer's; they also slow brain atrophy in early Alzheimer's.[36]	½ the daily dose with breakfast and ½ with supper	whole grains; dried beans; meat, fish, and dairy; fresh vegetables
omega-3: fish oil	Reduces inflammation and protects against heart disease, depression, and memory loss.	2000 mg omega-3 (or 1000 mg of DHA) daily	fatty fish: salmon, sardines, herring; nuts: walnuts, almonds; seeds: flax, pumpkin, chia, hemp
vitamin D3	Vital for immunity, mood, bone health, cancer protection, and glucose metabolism.	0–2000 IU daily April–October; 2000–5000 IU October–April (to raise vitamin D blood level above 40)	fish, eggs, fortified foods (like milk, orange juice, cereals); or 15 minutes of sun exposure 3–4 days per week
magnesium	Magnesium deficiency is common and linked with cognitive impairment. Magnesium improves memory and neurotransmission.[37]	preferred form for the brain: magnesium L-threonate, 144 mg daily (or 250–750 mg daily of magnesium citrate)	leafy greens and fruits; dairy; whole grains; nuts and seeds; beans and legumes
probiotics	Help restore normal gut microbiome; vital for immunity, mood, and metabolism.	30–60 billion live cultures; look for product containing 6–8 different strains	yogurt, kefir, sauerkraut, tempeh, miso, natto, kimchi
vitamin E	Slows the progression of mild to moderate Alzheimer's.[38]	400–800 IU of mixed natural tocopherols daily (up to 2000 IU daily if diagnosed with dementia)	avocado, nuts, leafy greens, sunflower seeds, wheat germ

Supplement	Why It's Important	How to Take It	Food Sources
curcumin	Reduces inflammation and insulin resistance, relieves depression.[39]	400–600 mg two to three times daily (standardized for 95% curcuminoids)	turmeric, the yellow spice in mustard and curries
phosphatidylserine	A natural lipid (fat) that may protect nerve cells and improve memory and concentration as well as mood.[40]	200–400 mg daily	soy lecithin, meat, or organ tissues
acetyl l-carnitine and alpha-lipoic acid (ALA)	Potent antioxidants boost energy and alertness; may slow progression of cognitive decline.[41]	500–1500 mg daily of acetyl l-carnitine; 150–600 mg daily of alpha-lipoic acid	l-carnitine found in meats; small amounts of ALA in leafy greens
ginkgo biloba	A herb shown to improve blood flow to the brain and slow memory loss.	60 mg twice daily (standardized to 24% glycosides or ginkgolides)	ginkgo tea

Ten Dietary Guidelines for a Youthful Brain

Now on to the guidelines: the following ten principles will help you nourish and protect your brain, cool down inflammation, improve your digestion, and even regulate the expression of your genes, whether or not you add supplements to your diet.

1. *Eat mostly whole foods.*

Mother Nature has perfectly packaged the information our bodies need to thrive; it's called a whole foods diet.

- Get as much of your diet as you can from foods still in their natural state (unprocessed, unrefined, unaltered in any way).
- Shop mostly at the perimeter of the grocery store; most of the processed foods are in the center aisles. Or better yet, go to a natural foods store, co-op, or farmer's market.
- Read the labels on packaged food. If you can't pronounce the ingredients, put it back on the shelf. It's not a natural, whole food.

2. *Eat a varied diet.*

Despite the abundance in today's grocery stores, our ancestors ate a much wider variety of foods than we do today. Variety helps ensure that you will get *all* the micronutrients you need, and it also gives your body a break from the same old foods so that you're less likely to develop sensitivities to them.

- Follow nature's example and eat seasonally, locally grown foods. For example, in fall/winter, eat more meats and fats, squash, soups/stews, and comfort foods (a nourishing high-protein diet); in spring, eat lighter foods with lots of fresh greens and sprouts (a cleansing low-fat diet); and in summer enjoy the abundance of fresh fruits and vegetables (a cooling high-carb diet).[42]
- Mix up the grains, and bring back some old standbys from years gone by, like buckwheat, quinoa, raw oats, barley, rye, millet, and brown and wild rice.
- Get out of the habit of eating the same foods every day— most notably wheat and dairy. Rotating such common foods (ideally by eating them every three or four days) may

allow you to enjoy them without some of the problems
caused by overexposure to them.

3. *Emphasize a plant-based diet.*

The healthiest diets from around the world all have this in common:
they include a large quantity and variety of fresh fruits and vegetables.

- Aim for six to twelve servings (or more) per day of fresh
  fruits and vegetables. That sounds like a lot, but it's not
  hard to do. Remember to look for a variety of bright colors,
  including green, yellow, red, orange, and purple.
- Every day, try to include at least one leafy green (such as
  kale, spinach, spring greens, chard) and one cruciferous
  vegetable (such as broccoli, cauliflower, brussels sprouts,
  cabbage, bok choy).
- Enjoy fruits in moderation; they contain fructose, so the
  sweeter, riper fruits (especially dried fruits) can spike your
  blood sugar. Fresh or frozen berries are a good choice.

4. *Get more healthy fats.*

We've been trained to think that fats are bad, yet some experts think
that our ancestors, who had far less inflammatory illness than we do
today, got more than two thirds of their calories from healthy fats. One
reason for today's obesity epidemic is thought to be the replacement of
fat calories with sugar and carbs. Brain cells rely on dietary fats to aid
in mood and memory, and most of us would do well to replace some of
our carbs with healthy fats.

- Emphasize omega-3 fats: fatty fish (sardines, herring,
  salmon), nuts (walnuts, almonds, pecans), and seeds (flax,
  hemp, and chia).

- Use olive (or avocado) oil as much as possible for salad dressing and for low-heat cooking. For high-heat cooking choose grape-seed or coconut oil, and try to limit the omega-6 oils (corn, soy, peanut, canola, safflower).
- It may be fine to eat *some* saturated fats: recent research suggests they do not cause heart disease. We still think it's prudent not to overdo them. Get your meat, eggs, and dairy from grass-fed, hormone-free, organically (and humanely) raised animals.

5. *Rethink protein.*

High-protein diets are popular these days (think Atkins or paleo), and food manufacturers are responding to the protein craze by adding it to snack bars and other processed foods. But new research says that high-protein diets (defined as more than 20 percent of calories from protein) during middle age (fifty to sixty-five) pose about as much health risk as smoking, with rates of cancer and diabetes four times higher than those on low-protein diets. But *after* age sixty-five, the findings suggest that protein actually *protects* against cancer, and researchers say you should then eat more protein, which may also prevent loss of weight and muscle mass.[43]

- Unless you are very physically active, most men need less than 80 grams of protein daily, and women need fewer than 60 grams. As a rule of thumb, one serving size of protein is about the size of the palm of your hand. For men, that would be roughly 20–30 grams, and for women about 15–20 grams of protein.
- You *can* get plenty of protein from vegetable sources alone: beans, legumes, whole grains, even green vegetables all have protein. And eggs give you a perfect protein with the

full complement of all the amino acids you need. (For comparison, a four-ounce serving of meat has about 30 grams of protein; one egg has 6 grams, and a cup of beans has 15 grams or more.)

- If you're drawn to a low-carb diet for health reasons, replace the carb calories with healthy fats rather than added protein. Consider a modified paleo diet: about a quarter of the plate is made up of protein, a quarter is starch, and half the plate is vegetables, with added healthy fats.

6. *Reduce sugars.*

Because of all the bad things sugar does to your brain, not to mention your waistline, cutting it back may be the most important dietary change you can make. But plenty of research shows that the sugar habit can be hard to break. If you're a sugar addict, treat the challenge with respect and go slowly, but do address it.

- Start by reducing or eliminating the most obvious sugar sources: soda, juice, and other sweetened beverages.
- Next take on your sweet tooth and cut down on baked goods and other treats. Most people don't have to eliminate them, just limit to once a day for starters, then a couple of times a week. Eventually you may want to save treats for special occasions.
- Finally, look for the less obvious sources of sugar, such as packaged foods (80 percent of them contain sugar), condiments, processed meats, peanut butter. Don't forget that breads and pastas made from refined flour are essentially the same as sugar. Also, it's best not to replace sugars with artificial sweeteners. They can be just as bad, or worse, for brain function.

7. Be good to your gut: get more fiber and probiotics.

Fiber won't keep you youthful if you otherwise eat a poor diet, but it sure helps. A high-fiber diet improves digestion and elimination, keeps weight down, slows sugar absorption, removes toxins, and feeds the good bacteria in your gut. Few of us get enough fiber *or* probiotics. Here's how to do it:

- Aim for at least 50 grams of fiber daily (most Americans get 20 grams or less). Fiber comes from the undigested parts of plants, so adding more vegetables and fruits as recommended above will help, especially if they are fresh and crunchy. Some of the best fiber fruits are berries, apples, and kiwi; high-fiber vegetables include peas, broccoli, and cabbage.
- The best dietary sources of fiber are beans and legumes, but if you aren't used to eating them, add them to your diet slowly (you know why). Whole grains are also good. And don't forget that nuts and seeds (flax, chia, and hemp) have a great deal of fiber. Many people also benefit from adding raw psyllium to their diet.
- Consume some kind of probiotic-rich food nearly every day. These include yogurt, kefir, fermented vegetables like sauerkraut, and several Asian foods (including miso, kimchi, and the drink kombucha). Be sure that they contain live cultures, and remember to aim for variety. You can find many kinds of fermented vegetables in food co-ops, or you can save money by fermenting your own.

8. Minimize toxins.

Toxic chemicals tend to gravitate toward fat, making brain cells especially vulnerable. You could do everything else perfectly, but if you let too many toxins into your body, all your efforts would be undone. It may not be possible to completely avoid toxin exposure, but whatever you can do will pay huge dividends.

- Buy organic foods if you can afford them. If you can't afford all organic, at least choose them when you buy produce that is most likely to be contaminated: the Environmental Working Group's "dirty dozen" (apples, celery, cherry tomatoes, cucumbers, grapes, hot peppers, nectarines, peaches, potatoes, spinach, strawberries, bell peppers, kale, and summer squash).[44] Also look into farmer's markets or community-supported agriculture groups (CSAs), where you can find good value on fantastic fresh vegetables.
- Limit your fish intake to once or twice a week. While the omega-3 is good for you, there is too much pollution in our waters. According to the Environmental Defense Fund, the safest choices (that are also environment-friendly) include arctic char, mackerel, wild Alaska salmon, rainbow trout, and US or Canadian albacore tuna.[45]
- Enjoy alcohol in moderation. Many studies suggest that a little alcohol can be good for the brain and may even reduce risk for dementia.[46] Red wine appears to offer heart benefits. But while a little may be good, too much is clearly bad. Men should limit themselves to two drinks per day, and women to one. More than that is associated with significant cognitive decline.[47]

9. *Flush your system.*
No matter how careful you are, you will still get some toxic exposure. Detoxifying the body ought to become part of your personal hygiene routine. This can be simpler than you may think.

- Everything works better when we are well hydrated, so be sure to drink plenty of pure water (plastic bottled water is *not* recommended, since plastic itself may contain toxins). Adding a little lemon makes it more detoxifying. Aim for eight or more twelve-ounce glasses per day: for example, two first thing upon arising, two more during the morning, two more in the afternoon, and small amounts of water with meals. Slow down in the evening to reduce nighttime trips to the bathroom.

- Reduce caffeinated and sweetened beverages. While they contain liquids, both caffeine and sugar can be dehydrating. Instead, drink more green tea (it contains minimal caffeine), or detoxifying herbal teas containing ginger, dandelion root, milk thistle, or peppermint.

- Consider an occasional or seasonal cleanse. They range in complexity but don't have to be too difficult to improve your digestion and help remove toxins from the body. See the Resources section for recommendations.

10. *Eat more mindfully.*

This could be a chapter in itself. The benefits of bringing more awareness into your relationship with food are enormous. Research shows that slowing down helps us eat less because we get a sense of satiety, more nutrients can be derived from our food, and there is less risk of obesity or diabetes. We believe that if you eat more mindfully, you will better know what your body really needs, which foods are nourishing and which are harmful, and when you have eaten enough. Here are some simple guidelines, but if you'd like to enter more deeply into the art of mindfulness, see the Mindful Eating Practice section below.

- Slow down. It can be as simple as that. Really chew and taste your food. Then chew some more.

- Pay greater attention to the act of eating, from start to finish: sensations of hunger, anticipation of the meal, the sight, smells, and texture of the food, and the mechanics of chewing, swallowing, and then going back for another bite.
- Notice when you first begin to feel satisfied; try to slow down even more, and when you feel you have had just enough, see if you can stop eating, even if there is more on your plate.

◇◇◇

A Helpful Practice
Mindful Eating

- Set aside a time to eat a meal alone or in silence with willing partners.
- Put some thought beforehand into what you want to eat. Since you will pay greater attention to the food, you may wish to choose more healthy, wholesome, and flavorful fare.
- Prepare the food with awareness and attention.
- Sit down, close your eyes, and allow the mind to quiet for a few moments. Give thanks for your food if you'd like.
- Engage all your senses: Look at the food, the shape, color, and amount of it. Smell it before putting it in your mouth. Feel the warmth, substance, and texture as you touch it to your lips and then place it in your mouth. Taste each bite, noticing how different the experience of taste is in different areas of the mouth. You can even listen attentively to the sounds of the body enjoying a good meal.
- Before you take your first bite, notice the feeling of hunger in your belly, the sense of anticipation, the changes occurring in your mouth as it prepares to receive the food.
- Pay special attention to that first bite, how vividly you taste it, how the tongue and entire mouth come alive.

- Chew each bite very slowly, resisting the urge to quickly swallow and move on to the next bite. Lightly hold the awareness of how you usually rush through the act of eating and scarcely even notice the food.

- Make each bite a deliberate act, one to be savored and enjoyed.

- Pay attention to the mechanics of eating, the movement of jaw and tongue, the way your body knows how to handle the food, chewing and moving it back toward the throat. Resist the urge to swallow until the food has been thoroughly chewed and the taste fully extracted. Then pay close attention to the act of swallowing itself.

- Continue in this way, returning to awareness of eating whenever the mind takes you somewhere else.

- Keep some of your awareness on your belly; notice especially when you are beginning to feel satisfied, as though you have had enough. See if you can stop eating *before* you have the sensation of fullness.

- Try to do this for at least part of each meal, and do it for an entire meal as often as you can.

Part 3

The Middle Way

Navigating between the Extremes for a Vibrant Mind

We can experience any kind of pleasure and pain either too much or too little. But to experience all this at the right time, toward the right objects, toward the right people, for the right reason, and in the right manner—that is the median and the best course, the course that is a mark of virtue.

—ARISTOTLE

In Buddhism, the Middle Way refers to the path to relieve suffering by learning to regulate one's thoughts, impulses, and behaviors. Aristotle's golden mean, from the Western philosophical tradition, offers a similar idea. It suggests that we should strive to find a mean between any two extremes of thought and behavior, given that each extreme represents a human vice. Both Eastern and Western philosophies recognize that any human characteristic could be a negative when expressed in its extreme, unregulated form, whereas a balanced, middle position of that same characteristic has positive virtues.

This section describes the *middle way of the mind*. This middle path develops essential abilities enabling a more fulfilling way of engaging life on its own terms. Cultivating the mind's capacity for the essential characteristics *curiosity*, *flexibility*, and *optimism* sustains the health of the brain and allows for the flourishing of the heart. These topics represent a bridge between physical practices that support the brain and the higher practices that connect us to others and to our highest potential for living with authenticity.

None of these essential characteristics develops automatically or in a vacuum. They are interrelated. Curiosity helps us to engage deeply with the world. Flexibility allows us to adjust and adapt to what we encounter along the way. Optimism enables us to persevere with hope and trust regardless of the obstacles we encounter. All three support our mental and emotional health as we age. The next three chapters provide the information and the concrete steps you need to develop these qualities, and yourself, to the fullest.

7

A Youthful Brain Cultivates Curiosity

Key 4

I have no special talents. I am only passionately curious.
—ALBERT EINSTEIN

Key Concepts

- Curiosity activates the reward centers deep within the brain.
- Curiosity is a whole brain exercise that integrates the knowledge circuits of the left brain with the pattern-seeking circuits of the right brain.
- Curiosity reboots the brain, keeping it fresh and vital by balancing knowing with a hunger to know more.
- People who find ways to express curiosity in their daily lives tend to have longer, healthier, and more fulfilling lives.

Does Curiosity Always Kill the Cat?

Here is a challenge for you. Read through the following word list and determine what mental characteristic they *all* suggest in common: *Restless. Distractible. Intelligent. Easily awed. Easily bored. Bold. Hun-*

gry. Daring. Mischief-making. Adventurous. Reckless. Content. Impulsive. Knowledge-seeking. Easily addicted. Socially gifted.

All these words describe personal characteristics that are strongly linked to the mind state we call *curiosity*. If you noticed a slight quickening of your pulse, if you felt compelled to solve this word puzzle, you probably rank high on the scale of this mental quality yourself.

Curiosity often involves a mild sense of uneasiness. When doing the word challenge above, for example, parts of your brain may experience it as unpleasant. But it is also a powerful motivator that can get us to pursue something, and we may experience great pleasure when we obtain it. Curiosity can also be quite fickle, leading us to explore something that grabs our attention in one moment, but then impulsively moving on to something else that glistens brighter in the next moment. Without the benefit of sustained attention, curiosity can be a source of distraction or mischief (think of the adventures of Curious George) or even danger. After all, didn't curiosity kill the proverbial cat?

Curiosity is related to an experience of dissatisfaction and discontent. Brain imaging studies confirm that mental states of curiosity may even share circuits with the mental state of depression![1,2] But the same feeling of discontentment that can be paralyzing to a person with depression may instead drive a curious person to explore new horizons. The brain's right hemisphere—so good at identifying new patterns of sensing, feeling, thinking, and behaving—links up with the brain's reward centers to convert an unpleasant experience into something deeply pleasurable.

That's what may have driven some of history's most famous curiosity seekers to such dramatic discoveries. Christopher Columbus, for example, was believed to have suffered from depression. But because there was such a strong activation of his brain's reward centers, his curiosity led him across the vast ocean to the discovery of a new world. Studies of present-day adventurers and risk takers show a similar mix of dissatisfaction with the status quo coupled with a motivated urge to find something better. Dissatisfaction, risk, and reward—these brain-based traits may drive the engines of curiosity, sometimes for the betterment of all.

Is Curiosity a Double-Edged Sword?

You can probably guess at the evolutionary purpose of curiosity. As with most evolutionary trends, it had a lot to do with survival. The simplest of organisms had little need for curiosity. When one's whole world is the ocean current that runs past your tentacles, like the enchanting sea anemone attached to coral reefs, there is little need for curiosity. The anemone only needs to sense whether there is food floating by in the current or whether the current is carrying something toward it that is dangerous. But as organisms got more complex, the development of curiosity became important. When they had to go forth and physically explore the world, to hunt or gather their food, animals needed a more sophisticated means of sensing and signaling what was happening in the world around them. Curiosity then became essential to survival.

It is worth remembering that curiosity sometimes *does* kill the cat. Too much curiosity can have devastating results, as many vivid examples from the animal kingdom illustrate. A baby hippopotamus wanders too far from its mother in a river also inhabited by crocodiles. The calf's curiosity borders on recklessness, and a river croc takes full advantage of it. He grabs the calf and holds her underwater long enough to drown her. The rest, as they say, is history.

Remember the tug-of-war between approach and avoidance that we discussed in chapter 2? This tension comes strongly into play in determining which people are driven by curiosity. At one end of the spectrum are those who avoid risk at all costs. At the other end are those fearless few who thrive on the excitement that comes from thrill seeking.

Studies of thrill seekers have shown that their brains are indeed different from other people's. In response to arousing images, their brains show much higher levels of activation by dopamine, often referred to as the pleasure chemical. Dopamine pours into their insula, a brain region where emotional signals from the body are processed and interpreted. At the same time their anterior cingulate cortex, an area involved with emotional self-regulation, is inhibited.[3] The accelerator is working, but the brakes are not!

This is the opposite of what happens for most of us, who steer clear of such experiences in favor of what is more safe, familiar, and predictable. The study concludes that people who crave high-risk, thrill-providing experiences have much stronger brain-based *approach systems*, while at the same time lacking the fear signals that would cause most of us to stop, turn, and run in the other direction.[4] They focus on what is exciting, intriguing, or attractive without being tipped off that with all the excitement comes inherent danger as well.

Returning to evolution for a moment, it makes sense that there is such a wide range in the degree of curiosity or thrill seeking among human beings. It would have been a big advantage for a tribal group to have some members who were willing to explore beyond their known world. That trait allowed ancient humans to gradually spread over the earth and survive in so many different habitats. But while you might want to have a *few* such individuals in your tribe, you would not want too many! Too much curiosity, too little braking power in the face of danger, and too little wisdom about risk versus reward would probably not be good for any group. As usual, nature has found a balance between extremes.

Evolution has devoted millions of years to finding the balance between survival-enhancing exploration and survival-threatening risk taking. The result is that modern humans exhibit a bell-shaped curve in their degree of curiosity. Some of us show just a bit, some an abundance, and most of us fall somewhere in the middle. There is no right or wrong, no good or bad in your own degree of curiosity. But there are some advantages to cultivating more curiosity as we age, and we hope to show how you can nudge your curiosity level just a bit higher to obtain the mental, physical, and social rewards that it offers.[5] By the way, you can do that without becoming a thrill seeker!

The Advantages of Ambiguity and Uncertainty

"I've never felt like this, but it's like I'm claustrophobic about my whole life." Up until that moment, at age fifty-two, Susan's life had followed a predictable routine established when her children were young. Now that they had moved on to college, and with her husband still highly engaged at work, she struggled. Rather than feeling free to explore opportunities she had postponed for twenty-five years, she felt stuck. Like many people who have not actively cultivated the curious side of their nature, Susan was gripped with fear of letting go of the familiar when curiosity came calling.

Curiosity is the state of mind in which we are driven to go beyond what we already know and to seek what is novel, new, and unexplored. Without regular activation of the brain's curiosity circuits, we can subtly settle into what is overly familiar, routine, and predictable—as Susan did. These are not bad things, but excessively predictable lives can lead to stagnation, a kind a mental stalemate that can leave you falling behind in the evolving adventure of your own life. Indeed, this may be one of the reasons so many people struggle early in their retirement. While it can be nice to leave the stress of work behind, the lack of challenge, stimulation, or novelty is sometimes a high price to pay.

Curiosity has many dimensions. One of the most important is *external* or *internal*. Is your curiosity evoked by something external, like the challenges you might find in your workplace, or is it an internal trait that does not depend on what is happening around you? Our focus is on helping you to cultivate an internally generated sense of curiosity, which is the kind of curiosity more strongly associated with positive health benefits throughout life.

Many people seek predictability because it brings them a sense of control over the uncertain world in which we live. Of course, there is nothing wrong with wanting a sense of control over your life. But research suggests that the growth of new brain cells is stimulated best by being exposed to what is new, unpredictable, and uncertain. Exposure to what we don't know or haven't faced before compels us to come up with new strategies and new solutions—and promotes a more adaptable and flexible brain.

There are many advantages that can come from intentionally stretching ourselves in this way. People with higher degrees of curiosity tend to have

- a longer life expectancy.
- reduced rates of dementia.
- more fulfilling and purpose-driven lives.
- more satisfying relationships.
- greater ability to form new friendships throughout life.
- a sense of themselves as being happier and more content.

Our goal is to show how you too can cultivate this mental flexibility in your life with a few simple activities. While we accrue knowledge and experience simply by virtue of growing older, curiosity does not increase automatically with the passage of time. The wise cultivation of curiosity requires practice, focused attention, and a willingness to seek out uncertainty and pursue the mystery of what it means to be fully alive.

As we age, the brain retains a great capacity for curiosity, but that capacity has to be exercised. Curiosity gives you a whole-brain work-out. When you expose yourself to what is new and unexpected, you have to weave together what you already know (centered in the left brain) with the integration of this new experience (centered in the right brain). If your mind is curiosity-driven, then your brain is contin-uously expanding, modifying, and reconstituting its network of neural connections. In short, the commitment to becoming a lifelong learner is an important factor in keeping the brain young and flexible.

Cultivating the Curiosity Garden

Researchers have found that people's curiosity varies in terms of the following characteristics.[6] Look over this list and rate yourself on a 5-point scale where 1 means you rarely if ever experience that aspect of curiosity and 5 means it is like the air you breathe, that you are perpetually curious:

- How *intensely* do you experience curiosity?
- How *frequently* do you experience curiosity?
- How *long* does the experience last?
- How *broadly* or widely do you experience curiosity across differ-ent settings?
- How *deep* does your curiosity go? Is it sustained even as you learn more about what made you curious?

Add up your scores. Do you fall in the highly curious range (18–25); a mod-est range (10–17); or in the minimally curious, easily satisfied range (less than 9)? This is not a scientific measure, but it can give you a sense as to whether curiosity is a core *internal* aspect of your identity, and it can help you to decide whether you'd like to plant more curiosity seeds in your garden and more ac-tively cultivate them as you grow older.

A gentle reminder: the learning that is driven by curiosity is not nec-essarily the type found in books or taught in classrooms! A curious mind pursues *sensual* learning—in other words, learning that involves regular stimulation of one or more of our five senses (smell, taste, touch, sight, and sound). A walk through a flower garden or along an ocean shore; indulging in a new cuisine composed of aromatic spices and foreign tastes; attending a musical concert or theater production; listening to a comedian's edgy act; taking an art class or learning to throw clay; or simply driving to a friend's house by following a different route with unfamiliar visual landmarks: all these are examples of *sensual* learning that flow from curiosity. And while they give you a whole-brain workout, they are in a sense *effortless*.

This Is Your Brain on Curiosity

What happens in the brain when we cultivate curiosity? There are several interesting studies that link curiosity to physical *hunger*, to the pleasure we get from good *humor,* and even to an appreciation of *beauty*. The connections among these three seemingly disconnected phenomena are not as far-fetched as they might first appear. Within our brains there is a powerful reward center, one that lights up with activity whenever we enter a new situation that is similar to one that rewarded us with pleasure in the past.

We all know physical hunger. When our blood sugar levels drop, sensors in our blood vessels signal the brain that it is time to eat. We call this signal *hunger*, and it activates areas deep within the brain as well as higher brain centers within the cortex. Together those centers create an *emotional* motivation that becomes impossible to ignore. The feelings get louder and more urgent until they eventually force us to seek food to satisfy our hunger. When we do, we are filled with great pleasure.

Physical hunger is just one of many hungers that we are driven to satisfy. The brain is hungry too, but what it craves is something new and interesting to feed its curiosity. Our pleasure center is activated when we eat a great meal. And it's also activated when we experience novelty, challenge, and the thrill of triumph in the face of uncertainty.[7] A lifestyle diet rich in such curiosity-driven experiences satisfies the brain's cravings.

It makes sense that we are driven to repeat that which has rewarded us in the past. But it is surprising to learn that these same reward centers become active when we think that we are going to be rewarded by something but that guess proves to be *wrong*! Being surprised by an unexpected result grabs the brain's attention even more quickly than being correct and getting the results we expected.

When the mind is caught off guard by something it didn't expect, the fact quickly catches our attention. We don't like to be disappointed, after all! The brain's attention and memory centers become active in order to figure out how to actually reach the promised reward. In effect, the brain shows a *hunger* to learn, especially when its power to predict a result gets teased, such as when your guess gets you "close but no cigar." When the correct solution to the mystery is finally revealed, such as through delivery of the unexpected punch line of a good joke, the experience is usually pleasurable.

The link between pleasure and new learning is important to help us understand the central role curiosity can play throughout life, and how it can even help us to survive to later life. Tucked away inside our discussion is the point that curiosity is *future-oriented*. Curiosity is always looking forward to our having an experience that hasn't happened yet. We may be curious as to whether something that happened in the past will happen again, or we may be drawn to something simply because it is entirely new and we want to discover what is going to happen. The essential value of curiosity is that since we can't fully understand or predict just how things will turn out, we need something to help us deal with all that uncertainty.

A Curious Mind in a Beautiful World

High levels of curiosity also enhance our ability to notice and appreciate beauty. But why should we care about that when it comes to maintaining a youthful mind? It turns out there is a biological advantage that comes from an experience of beauty, and the ability to recognize and cultivate beauty in our lives can actually help us as we age.

If you want to have a vital, healthy brain, nothing but good comes from encounters with that which we perceive as beautiful. Beauty activates our attention centers in a powerful way, and it encourages us to remain focused on the object of beauty for a long period of time. We might literally find it hard to turn away, as though the beautiful thing has temporarily captured us. As we stare (or listen, or focus on an aroma), our brain is heavily engaged in processing all the information coming our way. What we find beautiful is often a mix of what is vaguely familiar and what is new, but it is often perceived as though it were being seen "for the very first time." When we perceive beauty, dopamine's release in the brain's reward center keeps us focused, captivated, and engaged.

In fact, perceiving beauty activates the same circuits that are active when we are highly curious. In effect, perceiving beauty may be a biochemical correlate of curiosity. From that perspective, the practice of play and the experience of beauty exercise critically important brain circuits involving the capacity to sustain attention, to engage in problem solving, and to come alive in a world full of wonder.

Leonard Shlain was a surgeon whose curiosity led him to explore the relationship between the world of art and the world of physics.[8] Could there be two stranger bedfellows? But in fact, Shlain's research backed up the idea that the beauty we perceive in both art and science stimulates curiosity that keeps our brain vibrant. Shlain says, "Revolutionary art and visionary physics are both investigations into the nature of reality."[9] In the hands of a curious artist, art seems to go beyond old forms and peeks into the future for what can be but isn't just yet. Perhaps that is why cutting-edge art forms often create tension in the viewer. In other words, beauty is a form of curiosity that drives us to ask questions, to explore the unfamiliar, and to examine what isn't known or understood. In that way, beauty, like hunger, is future-oriented and serves as an important motivator to create our future by engaging it more deeply.

There is another, often neglected dimension to the relationship of beauty and curiosity that seems particularly relevant to aging well. We are all too aware that time is passing and that the end of our own time is coming. We have all heard the saying that it is important to "stop and smell the roses." But as we age, it seems to us that time accelerates, and we ask with sincerity, "Where did all the time go?" As the composer Hector Berlioz wrote, "Time is a great teacher, but unfortunately it kills all its pupils."

The perception that time accelerates is a consequence of our growing life experience. More and more of what we encounter each day seems like variations on what we have encountered before, meaning that it takes less mental energy to make sense of it. But as we begin to perceive our lives through the lens of habit, our actual life experience falls out of conscious attention. The particular experience we are having collapses into and merges with prior similar experiences. It no longer stands out on its own as a separate and unique experience linked to a particular place and moment in time.

Curiosity can help us counter the tendency for time to collapse into undifferentiated sameness. Curiosity keeps us fresh in part because it keeps twisting the old into something new and vital. Children can play the same game with each other day after day because to them, it is never the same game twice. The rules and experiences keep changing. Beauty too is a game changer. It exposes us to what we may have seen before but never in quite the same way. Beauty gives us feelings of vibrancy, vitality, and renewal. Who among us wouldn't want to experience those feelings on a regular basis, especially as we age?

Full of Wonder about What's Next

"'Curiouser and curiouser,' cried Alice . . . 'Oh, my poor little feet, I wonder who will put on your shoes and stockings for you now, dears?'"[10] While in Wonderland, where nothing was as it was expected to be, Alice found her body growing upward and becoming taller, leaving her feet far below her hands. Her comment, reflected in the very title of the book (*Alice in Wonderland*), highlights the link between curiosity and those aspects of our lives that have yet to completely reveal themselves. Alice knew she was facing a predicament that was strange, to say the least, but her thoughts already turned toward figuring out what she might do given the uncertain situation she found herself in.

This orientation toward the future is at the very core of what our brains are designed to do. Intelligence has been found to be less about what we know, our mastery of facts and figures, than about how effectively we are able to *predict* what will happen based on the information available to us. When we know just enough about something new to engage our attention and focus, curiosity provides the motivational drive to explore our environment (or ourselves!) so we can learn if we were right or wrong. When something is vaguely familiar or partially recognizable, studies show, brain areas involved in focusing attention and encoding new learning become more active *at the same time* that subjects in these studies report a *feeling* of curiosity.[11,12] Perhaps that is why there is such a strong correlation between intelligence and curiosity: an intelligent mind is often a curious mind, and a curious mind gathers new experiences that add to our storehouse of accumulated knowledge and wisdom.

When our clients come to us, it is often because certain problems in their lives have become so routine, so automatic, and so apt to occur without thinking, that the odds of coming up with a new solution to an old problem are quite low. Part of our therapeutic approach is to engage and activate our clients' curiosity to discover new solutions. It is often a hugely rewarding experience for people to discover a new resource within themselves or a new way of addressing a problem that has long resisted change.

The Curious Balance of Risk and Reward

We have already discussed the association between curiosity and reward. Obtaining a reward is often pleasurable. Our brain gets flooded with dopamine when we anticipate the reward we are about to obtain. It pushes us to work harder, to explore longer, to stay focused on the goal, and to strain to provide that last bit of effort to secure the reward. As soon as the reward is actually obtained, serotonin (dopamine's companion chemical in the brain's pleasure center) floods the brain. The feeling we experience is of being full and satisfied.

Serotonin is the *safety and satiety* molecule. It leaves us content and calm. As we said earlier, the feeling of satiety isn't restricted to satisfying food-related hunger. Curiosity drives us to satisfy many forms of mental and emotional hunger, and our primary reward—regardless of how long it lasts—is the chemically induced brain state of contented relaxation and comfort. Temporarily, we can curl up and enjoy a few moments under the calming influence of serotonin.

Unfortunately, this future orientation of the brain can get us into all sorts of trouble, as any compulsive gambler will attest. Compulsive gambling is an example of curiosity run amok. A compulsive gambler intellectually knows the odds of winning are small. But the gambler's rational mind is overcome by the combination of overstimulation of the brain's approach circuits and the understimulation of the inhibitory circuits. This push can lead to distortions in thoughts and emotions so that the gambler fails to recognize the danger of gambling beyond what he (or she) can afford. The line between entertainment and addiction gets crossed. Gamblers anticipate the possibility—or in their mind the *inevitability*—of winning, while any hope of applying their behavioral brakes fades until it is too late. Their financial losses may mount, but any wins along the way reinforce the conviction that the big score is in the next hand or the next spin of the roulette wheel. When the financial crash finally comes, as it almost invariably does, feelings of shock, remorse, shame, and despair explode. But for the compulsive gambler, those negative feelings soon fade and are replaced by excitement at the possibility of winning *even more* next time.

People who have a normal degree of curiosity can anticipate those negative consequences, enjoy some time at the casino, and stop before significant problems arise. For such people, gambling is an entertaining, enjoyable pastime, not an addictive and self-destructive habit. Their pleasure center still drives them toward something (that's the approach system working), but it also activates their avoidance system, and they can exercise better judgment by comparing current circumstances with memories of past experiences.

Curiosity, like every other capacity in the brain, has an upside and a downside. We need to practice moderation, exercising our judgment and wisdom while expanding our curiosity. Without curiosity, the brain as we age settles into sameness and allows the avoidance system to become dominant. The result is a life out of touch with novelty, growth, and the brain-enhancing benefits that come with being regularly challenged to adjust and adapt to an ever-changing world.

The Case for Boredom—in Moderation

We have seen how curiosity can be dangerous when it is not balanced with caution. Curiosity also needs to be balanced with a tolerance for boredom. As we age, it might seem as though we naturally move from youthful curiosity to boring routine. Studies distinguish between a state of temporary boredom and a chronic trait of boredom that is closely linked to depression.[13] No one wants to feel dulled or bored all the time, but transient feelings of boredom are an important counterpoint to unbridled curiosity. Developing a tolerance for sameness, the ability to take a mental, physical, and emotional pause, can protect us from perpetually chasing after what is new and appealing.

As the mind extracts the information from a new experience, there will come a point at which we will have gotten all the most useful morsels out of it. At that point, a feeling of emotional fullness sets in. That is the moment when transient boredom arises. We typically have one of two responses to that feeling of boredom. We can mentally push ourselves away from the table, refusing another bite no matter how tempting, because we want to digest what we have just taken in. That process of digesting what we have just consumed is critically important for encoding and consolidating experience. That processing makes the experience available in a useful way when we need to draw upon it in the future.

The alternative response is to shift our focus. Transient boredom tells us that there seems to be little more of value in the situation and it is time to move on to greener pastures. Either way, transient boredom cues our curiosity to turn inward as we absorb what just transpired, or to turn outward, with motivated desire, to explore new environments in the search for novel experience. A little boredom can be a good thing! Let's learn to tolerate and even embrace it.

Building Curiosity in the Second Half of Life

How do you learn the dance of curiosity? What are the basic steps? Based upon what we have looked at in this chapter, you may have guessed the basics. You may be right, or maybe you're not. You'll have to read on to discover how well your mind's prediction circuits are currently working.

Remember that we want curiosity to become something your

mind brings to your world each day, not simply a short-lived reaction to something new. The goal is for curiosity to become your habitual outlook on life, a natural feature of your worldview. To achieve that takes practice. You can start by deliberately planning activities that promise uncertainty and surprise. Think of curiosity as what leads you away from comfort through some temporary discomfort to an increased capacity for pleasure. What follows are suggestions for using curiosity to move outside your current comfort zones.

Slow Down to the Pace of Life

How many of you have said about an upcoming vacation that you are looking forward to "doing nothing except relaxing"? That may have been your innate wisdom telling you that you desperately need to get off the treadmill or risk burnout.

We are at risk of burnout when the pace and number of our daily activities have been too much for too long. Signs of burnout include physical exhaustion, loss of motivation, a loss of purpose or meaning, a growing cynicism or negative outlook toward others, and an inability to feel satisfaction or pleasure in what you do. When in a state of burnout, it is hard to generate curiosity because that involves seeking out even more stimulation. A vacation is designed to clear out the mental/sensory logjam, allowing you to once again take in new experiences. Of course, a weeklong vacation once every year or two is simply not enough time for people to fully restore their capacity for healthy curiosity.

The second half of life invites us to ask questions designed to prevent burnout. What is my true purpose? What to me has the most meaning? What do I need to live a life that is fulfilling and joyous? To answer those questions requires a pace of life that allows for taking in the new and learning from the old. Look at the pace of your life. Does it allow time for this rhythm?

A Helpful Practice

Finding the Rhythms of Life

Consider participating in the kinds of activities each week that provide you with the rhythm of doing and nondoing:

- Take a nightly walk after dinner.
- Start a journal to record thoughts about the day.
- Record your dreams; gradually, themes from your deeper mind will come to light.
- Develop a meditation practice.
- Attend a yoga class.
- Take dancing lessons.

These are slower, patient, mostly gentle activities that involve lots of repeated practice. This repeated pattern generates the mental room for creativity to grow. By the way, sitting in front of the television for hours each night is *not* on the list. It has been shown to overstimulate the brain, contribute to sleep problems, and ultimately make living a healthier-paced life more difficult!

Seek Novelty

Commit to regularly pursuing activities that take you out of your comfort zone of familiarity. Search for surprise. Do something unexpected and spontaneous. You will find that your comfort zone is likely to keep expanding. Do things with which you have little prior experience. The goal isn't to find something you'll necessarily fall in love with. Rather, it is for you to stimulate your senses by experiencing something that you hadn't even considered experiencing before.

Grow Your Novelty Skills

Think about expanding your comfort zone of competence. By engaging in activities that are just a bit beyond your current skill level, you will see your competence grow. The brain never loses its appetite for growth, and providing mental and physical challenges is an important way to satisfy the brain's hunger for continued growth. Passion and curiosity are effective counterweights to anxiety, worry, and fear. Curiosity expands the boundaries of your life, while anxiety and fear lead to mental, physical, and emotional constriction and confinement.

Here is a simple practice, a curiosity-building exercise that you can develop fairly easily. Get your hands on a copy of your community's paper that publishes upcoming events—free shows, art fairs, movie or theater premieres, restaurant openings, or other events new on the scene. Make the commitment to pursue two new events per month for the next three months. Following your participation in each event, ask yourself the following questions and keep a journal of your responses. The result will be a curiously expanded mind and an enriched life.

- In what ways was the activity similar to what I've done in the past?
- In what ways did the activity expose me to something new?
- What is something new I learned that I didn't expect?
- What did I discover about myself that I didn't recognize before?
- How can I apply this learning to other parts of my life?

◇◇

Learn to Enjoy Doing Things Independently

Strike a balance between those activities that you do on your own and other enjoyable activities that you can do with your friends. Doing things independently improves your relationship with yourself. You are an amazingly complex being and there is much about you to discover—an example of curiosity turned inward. As you become better acquainted with and more accepting of who you are, you can bring a more contented self to your interactions with others. In turn, this can make for deeper and more meaningful connections with them. If you are of a certain age and means, consider joining an Elderhostel program either alone or with a spouse/partner.

Engage in Regular Play

More about the importance of play will be found in chapter 11. For now, let's simply say that it is hard to find a more potent curiosity builder than free, unadulterated play. One of the characteristics of true play is that it is open-ended and not rule-bound. In fact, to watch children at play is to observe how the "rules" of their games keep changing any time they begin to become bored and lose interest. They instantly improvise new rules. Continuously modifying an experience so that the mind remains engaged is certainly good for the developing brains of children. And research has shown that the same holds true for the evolving brain of an aging adult.[14]

How do you have fun? When is the last time you did something for the sheer pleasure of it? Who or what makes you laugh the most? Answer those questions for yourself and then commit to obtaining a regular dose of play in your life.

A Curious Conclusion

There is an irony to closing out this chapter. A conclusion involves something coming to an end, whereas curiosity, as we've said, is very much about looking forward to new beginnings. So to review (which literally means to *re-view* or to look at once again), we will look back so you can look ahead to what comes next.

We have described curiosity as an outgrowth of our internal unrest. For some, that unrest generates the motivation to pursue new opportunities and new challenges. It is a potent and creative force. It can be a healthy blessing that helps to keep the brain vitally alive as it is continuously bathed in new experiences.

For others, curiosity represents a kind of perpetual discontent that has something in common with depression. It can be a feature of an unsettled mind and a disorganized life. We wish to strike a balance between healthy seeking and constant distraction, recklessness, or disillusionment.

Clearly, our bias is to learn how to harness the creative potential of a curious mind. Doing so involves embracing internal unrest and channeling it in new directions as you begin to forge a curious new path in your evolving life. As poet Robert Frost wrote,

> *Two roads diverged in a wood, and I—*
> *I took the one less traveled by,*
> *And that has made all the difference.*[15]

8

A Youthful Brain Stays Flexible

Key 5

People will try to tell you that all the great opportunities have been snapped up. In reality, the world changes every second, blowing new opportunities in all directions, including yours.

—KEN HAKUTA

Key Concepts

- Increasing our mental and physical flexibility as we age seems to run counter to nature's design, but that has more to do with fear than with destiny.
- Learning to respond more flexibly to change offers important benefits that may make life more enjoyable, rewarding, and fulfilling.
- Thinking about thinking, or *metacognition*, is an important brain-based ability for increasing mental flexibility with age.
- Cultivating *response flexibility* involves learning a manageable set of skills that simultaneously strengthen stress hardiness while reducing fear.

"My life is essentially finished." This outlook is all too common in the second half of life. Many people do not feel a sense of fulfillment or satisfaction about the completeness of their life. They are full of regrets about missed opportunities and a wishing for what might have been.

As we age, we are invited to reexamine, reevaluate, reenergize, and refashion how we live going forward. We have the opportunity to make conscious choices that will influence how we actually live. At some point, we all receive the invitation to enrich the quality of our lives. It is rare to go through life without hearing that call of an inner voice that challenges us to make changes to enrich our lives. Ultimately, the call is an opportunity to ask, "Am I aligning my life with the best in me so that I can offer the best to those around me?" But not all of us choose to invest the time and energy in exploring how to respond to that inner voice. What makes responding to the call so challenging?

- Fear of going beyond what we've grown comfortable with—feeling that the "devil we know is better than the devil we don't know."
- Avoidance of what seem like daunting challenges. Cultivating new paths for living can be hard work, even when our current path is clearly outmoded, emotionally spent, and spiritually unsatisfying.
- As we age, we are biologically less capable of making changes that would open up new possibilities for a more joy-filled and satisfying life *unless* we make the conscious decision to do so.

Watch Where You Put Your Mind

In chapter 2 we debunked the assumption that we inevitably grow less physically and mentally flexible as we age. We do become slower in our physical movements and slower to process certain kinds of *novel* information. But less flexible? Not necessarily. Older brains are sometimes able to process information with more flexibility than younger brains. Life experience has its benefits. Accumulated life experience provides a reservoir of variations and solutions that can be combined to increase options for responding flexibly. Older brains can be more efficient brains as a result. Neuropsychological studies of older subjects consistently show that retention of mental agility is to a large degree a function of attitude, practice, and experience, and not an inevitable consequence of time's passing.[1,2]

This brings us to the important influence of *premature cognitive commitments* (PCCs).[3] The brain is designed to learn and to convert learning into response patterns that quickly become automatic, unconscious habits. What we come to believe about our daily world reflects acquired biases of which we are scarcely aware, but these biases (PCCs) dramatically influence what we think, what we say, and what we do.

When we are exposed to information that we do not thoughtfully consider or critically evaluate, we unwittingly absorb and accept it. Advertisers make use of the ease with which we are influenced outside of our awareness. That is why we may suddenly sense that we *need* something we didn't even know we wanted! The role of PCCs is like what happens when we are infected by a virus that, unbeknownst to us, takes over a cell and directs it to produce new viruses. Similarly, our mind's belief systems are commandeered by PCCs to conform to their outlook without our awareness that it is happening. For example, we carry a wide range of cultural biases about aging that are faulty or even flatly wrong. Unexamined beliefs about aging reflect PCCs that influence our expectations to the degree that our daily functioning actually changes to conform to these false beliefs! Here are common examples.

- Getting older means getting sicker and more infirm before ultimately dying alone.
- Getting older means becoming a burden on everyone else.

- Getting older means you will get Alzheimer's disease and forget your loved ones.
- Getting older means becoming irrelevant and useless.

These negative PCCs, implanted outside of awareness, represent a major threat to the chances of our remaining flexible as we age.

Of course, we can also be infected by *healthy* biases and PCCs. Harvard University researcher Ellen Langer discovered this effect in studies in the late seventies and early eighties. In one study, she transported two groups of older adults to an isolated monastery where they stayed for a number of weeks. One group was asked to act "as if" they were younger versions of themselves. They were helped out by books, newspaper articles, old-time radio programs, and black-and-white television, all associated with the year 1959.[4] The second group was asked only to reminisce about those earlier years, to nostalgically think back but not necessarily act the part. By the end of the first week, the first group showed how much mental attitudes impact physiological and cognitive functioning.

The first group of adults had clearly "regressed." They broke out of their PCCs and showed measurable changes consistent with "growing younger." They were more physically flexible. A number were even playing touch football by the end of the week. Even more dramatic were the findings that their memory, the degree of gnarling in their arthritic fingers, the fluidity of the movement of their muscles and joints, and their intellectual functioning all improved. As Dr. Langer concluded, "Wherever you put the mind, the body will follow."

Flexible Coping When Nothing Stays the Same

The lessons of Langer's studies have been known for more than thirty years. The findings have been duplicated by others.[5] Why, then, are we still victims of premature cognitive commitments and the distorted perceptions they create? In a word, *fear*. When we function under the influence of the many forms of fear, we tend to become more rigid and less able to respond with adaptive flexibility. Instead of being able to thoughtfully consider, *Hm, what makes sense to do right here, right now?*, we respond out of fixed, preconceived, and automatic habits (those darned PCCs). Responding out of unconscious habit is the essence of a rigid response style.

We are actually designed for flexible responding. That is what has made the human species so adaptable and successful. But being flexible depends on active management of fear. There are differences in how people cope with fear and anxiety. Coping styles can be boiled down into two contrasting but complementary approaches, protective coping and adaptive coping.[6]

When under the influence of fear, the brain's prefrontal cortex (PFC), which helps us with higher-level thought and reasoning, is largely off-line. As a result, we revert to what we've known from our past, and that's usually our preset response patterns. So rather than responding more adaptively to the actual situation at hand, we hunker down in protective coping mode. Did you ever deal with your concern about a looming deadline by escaping into a movie rather than digging into the project? This kind of avoidance is a classic protective coping. A protective coping style is less flexible, more impulsive, more aggressive, and less attuned to the specific details of the source of stress.

Protective coping is influenced by the relative levels of dopamine and serotonin released by the brain: too little serotonin release and we revert to protective coping. Serotonin promotes calmness and contentment (one reason it is widely affected by antidepressant medications). As we age, serotonin levels naturally decline. So the protective coping style can then become the *default* style, resulting in more rigid, reactive response patterns. If we're not careful, our declining serotonin levels and increasing propensity for protective coping can actually make us less flexible in how we face life's challenges as we age.

But protective coping isn't inevitable. The converse is an *adaptive* coping style, and it can be learned and cultivated—at any age. An adaptive coping is slower, more thoughtful, and more flexible. It allows us to adjust and adapt to the specifics of the situation at hand, and possibly craft a more effective strategy for solving a problem that's in front of us.

By slowing down our response, adaptive coping allows us to attend to the details in a situation, and that means we can generate a tailor-made response—one that is likely to be more effective. In order to find this response, we must have the ability to pay focused attention to an issue and to sustain that attention over time. Adaptive coping takes more time, but the results permit greater adaptive flexibility.

Nobel Prize laureate Daniel Kahneman describes the interplay of these two systems of thinking and coping in his important book *Thinking, Fast and Slow*.[7] The slow thinking, adaptive system of coping relies on the release of dopamine, the attention-focusing molecule. Flexible coping requires the brain to be able to distribute *both* serotonin and dopamine effectively. Staying calm and focused can be very useful when creating new solutions to old problems. Therefore, simple practices that promote mind-brain health generally can also promote greater response flexibility throughout life. Some of the best practices are also the simplest. Common examples include

- learning to meditate.
- getting consistent and restful sleep.
- participating in activities that you enjoy and that challenge your mind.
- engaging in playful activities that regularly make you laugh.

- identifying what situations you find most stressful and disturbing while also developing a personalized plan for effectively managing your stress response.

Modern life demands adaptive coping. Without it, we can succumb to physical, mental, and emotional risks that increase as we age. But by taking active steps to promote optimal mind-brain health, we can face life with more flexibility and joy.

Fear, Fear, Go Away, Come Again Another Day

The pervasiveness of fear is nothing new. Chapter 2 of the Bhagavad Gita, the ancient Hindu text written at least 2,300 years ago, tells us, "No step is lost on this path, and no dangers are found. And even a little progress is freedom from fear."[8] To be flexible requires loosening our grip on what has been before so that we can open up to what comes next. Letting go requires that our hands are sufficiently open so that we can use them to construct the second half of our lives with a forward-looking, flexible plan, rather than anxiously glancing back over our shoulders as our "good old days" recede.

As the Gita says, even a little progress is freedom from fear. Small steps can make big differences. Twenty years ago a colleague named Bill wanted to go skydiving. When the day arrived, he was full of excitement. His more experienced skydiving friend Stan accompanied him, offering plenty of encouragement to calm Bill's nerves. When it was his turn to jump, Bill found himself on the platform to exit the plane, tightly gripping the handrail for dear life. Bill told Stan, "I can't let go!" Stan, wise and unflappable, calmly said, "That's okay. Don't let go. But surely, you can loosen just your index finger and hold on with the others." Bill agreed and did so. Next Stan said, "I'll bet you can hold on with just your thumb, your middle finger, and your pinky." Again, Bill agreed and discovered he could still hold on. When Stan pointed out that "it would be interesting to notice what happens when you're just holding onto the rail with the pinky and thumb," Bill loosened the middle finger's grip and, with only a thumb and pinky to hold him, found himself airborne. The free fall was exhilarating. The opening of the parachute occurred right on cue. The surreal descent back to earth was gentle. It was a giddy lesson in acquiring flexible learning, one simple step at a time.

Remaining Flexible in an Ever-Changing World

We are hardwired for fear. We are also hardwired for flexibility. Learning to cultivate a successful balance between our biologically based flexibility and fear-based rigidity helps us adjust and adapt to the challenges of the second half of life. There are many reasons why differences in flexibility show up across individuals (and often within the same individual!) over the span of their lives. The combination of our inborn neural wiring and our accumulated life experience creates what Michael Merzenich, the godfather of neuroplasticity research, describes as our "soft-wiring." In other words, we have genetic predispositions for fear or flexibility, but our brains are forever being modified by ongoing experience.[9]

Neuroplasticity is the ability of our brain to adapt and change—in effect, to be rewired. But how does that actually happen? Once a new response pattern is recognized and learned, and once the brain finds that this new pattern actually *works* to achieve a goal, satisfy a need, or solve a problem, the brain seems to let out a big neurological sigh.[10] Harmonious brain wave patterns reemerge. Deep within the brain's circuits, sweeping neuroplastic changes are under way.[11,12]

The rewiring brain sends out signals for new proteins to be synthesized. Instructions for genes to be turned on or off are received.

Chemical changes at the synaptic junctions linking one neuron to the next are catalyzed. The new way to get something accomplished gets encoded as a new neural firing pattern. This is the heart of flexibility. With time and repeated practice, the new way will morph into the old (established) way of doing things. At the same time, the aging but *youthful* brain maintains its search for something new to learn. And so, the tug-of-war continues between your being a lifelong learner and your being a security seeker, content with what you already know. Mind-body practices balance that tension.

Our neurobiology is designed to turn the unfiltered chaos we perceive through our senses into predictable and controllable routines and habits as quickly as possible. Not having to figure everything out for the first time is a major time saver. More important, it conserves precious metabolic energy that can mean the difference between survival and oblivion for most species. We don't have to take time each morning to figure out the best route to take to work. That learning is encoded and can be simply reactivated and downloaded into our routine each morning as we step out our front door. Those routines help to make life manageable by giving us a sense of predictability and control.

The reality, however, is that life *is* ultimately unpredictable and minimally controllable. Dr. Ken Druck, a renowned psychologist, had a seemingly ideal professional and personal life until the day in 1996 when he experienced a tragic loss. His beautiful daughter had been killed in a road accident while studying abroad. He says that in that instant, the tragedy "ended my life as I knew it."[13] Over time, his loss led him to look more deeply at life. He developed a set of "rules" or principles by which life can be lived more fully, despite our limited control over many of its unforeseeable twists and turns (specifically, he learned that a *breakdown* can lead to a *breakthrough*). Those principles are outlined in his book *The Real Rules of Life*. The rules guide us to respond with courage to what daily life often entails—how life actually *is*—so that we can learn to adapt and respond in order to create what we would like life *to eventually be*. This is the essence of flexibility.

Seeking flexibility requires tolerating uncertainty and ambiguity. Flexibility emerges from trial-and-error strategies of problem solving without knowing what the result will be, and such experimentation with new patterns of living is at the heart of curiosity. This search pattern often generates anxiety or even psychological upheaval. Lev Vygotsky, the early-twentieth-century pioneering Russian psychologist, introduced the idea that child development proceeds along a path that involves evolution and revolution. It is anything but a straight line of gentle, predictable growth.

He might as well have been discussing the challenge of remaining flexible in our approach to the second half of life. Having to adjust and adapt to change demands the ability to modify what we know and expect as we engage what is new and unfamiliar. Many people seek to avoid such changes by constructing a life of familiar and safe routines that keep anxiety (a mental form of fear) at bay. The price of overrelying on such efforts is to risk stagnation, and stagnation correlates with measurable shrinking and thinning of brain tissues, resulting in a clear loss of adaptive flexibility. In effect, our fear-driven beliefs about what we might become turns into the biology of who we actually are.

Natalie had a life crisis that demonstrates the frightening tension between the new and the familiar, and the capacity for neuroplastic change. Until her early fifties, Natalie's beauty defined her relationships. When her husband's serial infidelity came to light, so did her tremendous anxiety. Her fear-driven beliefs said that she could not survive outside the marriage. The well-rehearsed beliefs took their toll on her biology: she looked sallow, with limp hair, aching muscles, and intestinal and heart symptoms. She couldn't think straight! Fear-driven stagnation was pushing her to stay in old patterns. Through focused mind-body therapies, the forces of adaptability won out. As she broke free of the stagnating beliefs about her beauty, her anxiety gradually receded, right along with the biological symptoms that were the physical sign of the loss of adaptive flexibility.

By choosing to embrace uncertainty, we ready ourselves to explore the unknown. As we experiment with new ideas or activities, there arrives a moment when we finally gain a sense of competence, maybe even mastery. But until that magical moment, there is effort, frustration, and even impatience or irritation. The reward for pursuing flexibility is the moment when we can play the scales on the piano as though the fingers know what to do all by themselves, or when we develop the sales plan for a new customer without staying up all night writing it. These different experiences reveal that what had been a struggle begins to feel more natural, less exhausting, and even rewarding or inspiring.

The brain also has an insatiable appetite for continuing to learn—throughout life. It tires of stale routines and craves new learning that challenges us to grow. That striving for novel experience pushes us toward what is unknown, unfamiliar, and uncomfortable. We can even see this process on EEG readings of the brain's electrical activities. When we're engaged in something new, brain wave patterns initially become chaotic. Energy expenditure increases. Blood flows into the brain centers engaged in generating a new response. Sugar metabolism increases to feed those brain areas busily brainstorming new solutions to new problems, or inventive solutions to old problems. The brain is working hard to discern an identifiable pattern that can eventually turn into a repeatable habit.

Creativity, Innovation, and the Brain's Metronome

Becoming more flexible is not a straightforward process. Some of the steps are quite unexpected. Jazz is a musical genre known for in-the-moment innovation. It doesn't follow a set score, although the musicians repeatedly return to the basic musical theme, before setting off again on another variation. The creative tensions between the main melody and the improvisational sets define the wonder of jazz. Pianist Dave Brubeck said, "There's a way of playing safe, there's a way of using tricks, and there's the way I like to play, which is dangerously, where you're going to take a chance on making mistakes in order to create something you haven't created before."

Brubeck captured an important point that is relevant to becoming more flexible in our thinking and behavior. Risk is a necessary ingredient of the creative process. Logic suggests that people who are more creative have more flexible minds. How else do they come up with such mind-bending innovations? Surprisingly, research suggests just the opposite: that creativity and innovation *decrease* as response flexibility increases. Creativity needs to be balanced by the ability to ignore distractions and diligently persevere with the creative task, or it often fails to produce finished works. In other words, creativity flourishes when accompanied by the ability to maintain a fixed and prolonged mental focus.[14] This is one of the most important benefits of learning mindful attention skills, as discussed in chapter 3. Learning to focus on one thing, like one's breathing, opens the door to thinking more creatively about many things.[15] Like a metronome, a flexible mind sets the pace for the back-and-forth movement between novelty and familiarity, and between ambiguity and certainty.

Andrea Griffin of the University of Newcastle, Australia, in a study of mynah birds, showed that within that species, certain birds are more innovative but less flexible, adapting to their environments more gradually and cautiously. Other birds are more flexible, exploring their environments slowly but with fine attention to detail.[16] Some birds see "the forest" while others see the individual "trees." Her conclusion is that each ability is better suited for certain environments and certain circumstances. Most birds have both, but individual birds, like individual people, tend to fall along a continuum between rapid, inflexible, big-picture thinking and slower, adaptable, more detail-oriented thinking.

Innovation involves a kind of rule breaking. It often challenges established tradition, just as creativity involves "going where no one has gone before." Innovation and creativity are important when an individual encounters a new environment. Our ancestors would have faced this challenge over and over as they migrated to new climates and populated the earth. They had to scout a new environment by learning its features and identifying its resources and dangers. They had to delay implementing old ways as they determined what the new environment would require of them. Once the clan was established in the new environment, a different set of skills was needed. They relied less on adaptive flexibility and more on the ability to quickly apply what had been slowly and patiently learned. Details were less important. Rapidly applying more general rules and routines now became favored, and those most able to do that were often the most adaptable.

Which mynah bird are you? Are you drawn to what is shiny and new? Do you yearn for what is familiar and comforting? Knowing where along the continuum you tend to fall can provide you with an important clue on where to focus as you grow your flexibility. If you are a person who chases new experiences, the key is to become more comfortable with, and tolerant of, routines and repetitions. For that person, it is important to build "depth" by going deeper into an experience and staying with it for a time. On the other hand, if you are a seeker of sameness, the goal is to increase "breadth" of life by broadening the range of experiences you sample, even if the conclusion is that what is new *in this particular instance* is not to your liking. Different strokes for different folks. But response flexibility involves regular sampling of "strokes" from beyond your comfort zone.

Talk amongst Your Selves

An old *Saturday Night Live* routine featured a gabfest among different characters. Inevitably, the main character would become emotionally overwrought. Then she'd encourage the others to "talk amongst yourselves" as she worked to regain her emotional composure. When it comes to learning to be adaptive, flexible, and optimistically forward-looking, being able to "talk amongst yourselves" is vitally important. The difference is that all the "selves" are different facets of your own mind, and learning to have them talk together is a critical step in becoming an adaptively flexible adult.

How do you talk amongst your mind's inner selves? How do you begin? In *The Power of Habit*, author Charles Duhigg says that we may have little control over what triggers the habits that control our lives. Falling into old habits in spite of sincere resolutions to change can leave us feeling powerless. Certain people seem to set us off in predictable ways. Seeing that fast-food shop on our drive home from work can overwhelm our earlier commitment to go home, change into our exercise clothes, and head for the gym.

Duhigg also indicates that we may have little control over the reward a habit offers. While some of those rewards are chemical—the effect of alcohol, a wedge of chocolate, or a drag on a cigarette—others are more subtle but no less powerful (the compliment paid, the argument avoided, the recognition received, and the exposing of personal vulnerability dodged). It is the sequence of actions we take (the routine) that perpetuates the belief/habit that we lack the ability to alter our lives. Instead, like the jazz musician playing the same song, *only differently*, we can learn to introduce life-expanding flexibility into our daily routines, step by subtle step, until we have created a new repertoire of patterns, routines, and experiences that are more enriching and fulfilling.

◇◇

A Helpful Practice
Four Steps for Developing Adaptive Flexibility

Step One:

Minding the Body to Message the Mind

It is hard to deny our fascination with our physical body. We exercise it. We expose it to exotic and unsustainable diets. We surgically and irreversibly modify it. We take mounds of pills to cure it or cleanse it. We are either depilating it or seeking to replace the hair that used to grow on it. We color it, dye it, and tattoo it. And yet, for many of us, we also shame it with all sorts of messages about how it fails to look or do what it should in order for it—and for us—to be acceptable. Some of the most powerful messages we carry involve our aging body.

For centuries, it has been said that the history of a person's life can be read by looking at that person's body. For too many, that history would be a tale of resistance to time's advance. There is often a desperate urge to turn back the clock. We may have given up on being able to influence our future, so as time marches on, our sense of defeat gets more deeply etched into the body.

Many wisdom traditions have found that the most fundamental path to changing one's outlook on life begins not with the mind, but with careful attention to the body (see chapter 4). The goal is not to perfect the body but to learn to attend to its needs for nourishment, for stimulation, for pleasure, for rest and relaxation, for activity, for growth, and for love. Yoga, for example, can be a lifelong journey to the core of what matters most in our lives. Our body supports our most central mental, emotional, and spiritual needs. While yoga is wonderful, it isn't necessary for developing increased adaptive flexibility. Go for a nightly walk after dinner. Get a monthly massage. Join a Silver Sneakers class at the local YMCA. Join a birding club. Take swimming lessons. Ride a bicycle along a well-kept bike path. The choices are endless. The key is to engage in an activity with attention to the activity as well as to how the body *feels* while engaged in it. The important point is that by making these kinds of healthful choices, you are not only mending your body, you are taking an important step toward maintaining your mind in a youthful manner.

Step Two:

I Think It, Therefore I Become It

The ability to be aware of what you are thinking *as you think it* is called *metacognition* (also known as *mindfulness of thought*). Its companion is *behavioral self-regulation*, or the ability to modulate your moods and your behavior to best match the context in which you find yourself. Together, they are central to learning flexibility in your daily life. You may become anxious as you witness changes in your work world, the declines or death of aging parents, or the extent to which adult children move on, becoming immersed in the details of their own daily lives. These normal changes induce feelings of being both vulnerable and increasingly expendable.

Learning simple mind-body techniques to actively monitor your thinking is vital. Listening in on your own mind (while gradually inserting more balanced and self-compassionate thoughts) is a portable, powerful, and readily available skill. Monitoring or observing your thoughts is far different from debating them. Ironically, directly challenging or dismissing worries only serves to strengthen them. Practicing mindful awareness lets you observe your thoughts from a dispassionate, nonjudging position. With practice, this approach undermines and then dismantles the premature cognitive commitments (PCCs) we have all unwittingly absorbed. Replacing old PCCs with enlightened thoughts more flexibly suited to the potential of the second half of life turns on the brain's central regulator—the prefrontal cortex (PFC). This effectively soothes the fear-generating part of the brain. The more creative and innovative parts of the mind can then become engaged. What emerges are plans of action that may successfully counter the negative conversations that chatter away in most people's minds. Moreover, these practices help to direct and regulate behavior in ways most consistent with your values and ideals.

What isn't initially obvious is that these practices actually rewire your brain. In many respects, the brain is an equal opportunity consumer. If we feed it shaming, self-limiting, fear-generating messages, it absorbs them. If we feed it more positive messages about physical vitality and mental or emotional vibrancy, it absorbs them instead. The brain is the most complex, self-organizing system in the known universe. That complexity is a blessing that flowers when you use it to live the life you set out to live in your later years.

Here is a simple acronym to drive home how metacognitive or mindful practices lead to behavioral self-regulation, and how both can lead to greater response flexibility. Alan Marlatt, a professor of psychology, coined the acronym SOBER. We usually associate the word with abstinence from alcohol or drugs. Being *sober* also means achieving a quiet state of mind that is free from excess or extravagance, as in someone who is able to exercise effective self-control. Here are the five steps to a SOBER mindfulness practice.

Stop: Use mindful awareness to pause before acting on a thought; just pause.

Observe: Observe the thoughts and feelings you are experiencing without judging them.

Breathe: Take a few slow, deep, and calming breaths (to bring your PFC online).

Expand perspective: Engaging your PFC, take a big-picture view of your situation.

Respond wisely: Practice flexibility by selecting the response that is most consistent with your best self.

Step Three:
Build Empathy with Your Friend, ToM

Mindfulness practice is essential to developing greater response flexibility by helping us stand witness to our own thoughts and feelings. This puts us in the pivotal position of being able to influence those thoughts and feelings, and to then witness the impact this influence has on the thoughts and feelings that come next. Still, mindfulness is only half of a dynamic duo of sorts. The other half is called *theory of mind (ToM)* and is the basis of empathy (which will be the focus of chapter 10). Empathy is the social glue that emotionally connects us to one another. Brain-based ToM circuits are the seeds from which empathy grows. When we feel connected to someone, through empathy, we can feel emotionally safe and more secure. And often, the safer we feel, the more able we are to take the necessary risks that develop greater response flexibility when called upon to do so.

Almost all people possess at least minimum levels of empathy, which is partly how we are able to become couples, raise children, interact with co-workers, and do passably well in our various social relationships. In the second half of life, well-developed empathy skills enable us to respond flexibly as we interact with our aging peers, our children and grandchildren, and our larger community. Offering our accumulated wisdom while continuing to be open to learning from others and from a world that is rapidly changing around us rests on well-developed empathy abilities.

Empathy skills emerge from the same soft-wired brain as all the other skills we have identified. Therefore, like those other skills, empathy can be improved with gentle, repeated practice. Strange as it may seem, growing empathy toward others can be enhanced by becoming more sensitive to your *own* feelings first. Research has shown that the only way we know what someone else may be feeling is by being able to tune into the feelings inside ourselves that are generated by our interactions with them. In other words, we read the feelings we have in *us* to clue us in on what they are feeling inside of *them*.

Growing your empathy skills requires three steps, summarized as Stop, Look, and Listen. As people age, there is evidence that the ability to take another's perspective declines right along with other aspects of flexibility. But as Dr. Pam Greenwood[17] and others have pointed out, many of these changes are not inevitable consequences of aging, but rather the consequences of *not* continuing to exercise the abilities we have: we "use it or lose it." So, what is involved with exercising Stop, Look, and Listen skills?

Maintaining good empathy skills requires putting the mental brakes on our impulses. When you have a strongly negative emotional reaction, for example, you *lose* flexibility if you get swept up by the power of the reaction. If you don't put on the brakes, the emotion drives an inflexible response.

STOP: When the urge to react rises up, stop and create a momentary pause— a mental time-out—in the reaction cycle. Inserting a small mental space created by the stop allows the chance to look inside.

LOOK: What are you reacting to? What is your reaction linked to? Can you take a moment to regain your emotional composure and bring your mindfulness skills back online? Then, with the emotional freedom that comes with putting the brakes on runaway emotions, you can direct your empathic attention to them and listen to the other person.

LISTEN: What seems to be driving their behavior? Can you better understand where *they* are coming from so you can better respond to them with your best self leading the way?

This three-step process exercises empathy skills so that pausing, checking in, and tuning in to the other person becomes more automatic, rewarding you with greater response flexibility and deeper connections to others.

Step Four:

Write Another Chapter in Our Never-Ending Story

One thing that makes mysteries so enticing to read is our inability to predict how the story ends. The twists and turns that a good mystery writer weaves into the tale keep us guessing. One of the dangers of premature cognitive commitments is that they convince us that we know where our unwritten future will lead. We recognize that at some point our life will end. But if we believe we already know that our journey into the second half of our life will play out negatively or in an unsatisfying or unfulfilling way, we lose our motivation to actively influence the unfolding of that journey.

Imagine going to the airport for a scheduled flight. You find your seat, put your bag into the overhead bin, buckle yourself in, and wait for the flight attendant to go through the usual preflight monologue. Only this time, it is an invitation to a dialogue. The flight attendant says, "Welcome aboard," and then asks, "Where would you like to go today?" How would you answer the question? Are you even *prepared* to answer the question? And since life is more about the journey than the destination, what if the question were about the particular path you want your life's inner and outer journey to follow?

It is said that human beings do not exist outside of their story: a personal narrative that ties together their various experiences, memories, and dreams into a coherent whole. What is often overlooked is that the story is being actively constructed by us throughout our lives, not dictated to us from some prewritten script. Living in a way that recognizes that we are the writer, producer, director, and central actor in the narrative story that we write is not easy, especially when we have forty, fifty, sixty or more years of remembered history that can seem so compelling. We can easily forget that it is never too late to make essential changes to the narrative script of our lives.

Here are questions to help you become an active author of the untold story that is the rest of your life.[18] 1. Get a tablet of paper and write down what you most want out of your life. 2. Then consider what you write in terms of how *invested or committed* you are to obtaining what you seek. 3. Next, ask yourself how *challenging or difficult* it will be to reach your goals. 4. Finally, ask yourself how *desirable* the goal is and in what ways it might be *rewarding*. Then, after getting an idea of what you are after, ask yourself the following questions:

- What are the actions you are actively taking that are intended to reach the goals you have set?
- With unblushing honesty, consider whether what you are doing is working. Is it bringing you any closer to your goals?
- How are the goals you have set, and the steps you are taking, making a positive impact on you and on the world around you?

- When you imagine yourself in the future continuing to act in a way consistent with the path you have identified, what are the feelings that you experience now?
- If five years from now someone who knows you well wrote a single paragraph about you, what you do each day and how you conduct yourself and impact your community, what would the paragraph say?

Rewriting the history of your future helps you increase your adaptive flexibility. Are you ready?

◇◇

9

A Youthful Brain Is Optimistic

Key 6

The US Constitution doesn't guarantee happiness, only the pursuit of it. You have to catch up with it yourself.

—BENJAMIN FRANKLIN

Key Concepts

- Optimism is hardwired into our brain as a skill that can be increased with practice.
- Optimism evolved to keep us engaged even when logic suggests we give up.
- Optimism is related to hope, trust, faith, and madness.
- Higher levels of optimism lead to measurable physical and mental health benefits.
- Optimism supports greater resiliency in the face of age-related challenges and setbacks.

Optimism and Its Closest Relative

Consider the courage it takes to face our common future. We know we will not live forever. Our lives will end at some point. We witness the passing of friends and family. The older we get, the more common an experience this becomes. Older adults report a sense that time is accelerating. We experience the effects of time's passing in our physical bodies. Formerly simple activities can now stretch out time, taking longer to organize, initiate, and complete. These are inescapable truths. They are inevitable and unchangeable. But our response to their challenges is not. As Benjamin Franklin reminded us, our task is to "catch up" with happiness. Balanced optimism, as this chapter shows, is a core element in the spirited pursuit of happiness, especially in the midst of the challenges of a time-limited life.

To face the realities of the second half of life with courage, joy, and wonder is the essence of optimism. Optimism requires a leap of faith. Optimism involves seeing into the future as it could be, and then acting in ways that bring that imagined future to life. Quite often, optimism requires boldness and daring to overlook current realities that dim the odds of achieving future goals. As playwright George Bernard Shaw once said, "Some men see things as they are and ask why. Others dream things that never were and ask why not." Some people dismiss such ideas as sentimental. Optimists, however, are not just romantic dreamers.

Neuroscience researchers have found that optimism enables us to persist in our efforts to generate a more positive future in spite of or even because of current obstacles and setbacks.[1] Biologically, it means that when the going gets tough, the optimists keep going! In that sense, optimism is our engine for the growth, exploration, and progress that have shaped the modern world. In short, optimism is related to faith, trust, and hope. It is also a cousin of delusion and madness. That is why the focus of this chapter is on balanced optimism.

Keeping the Faith—with Persistent Hope

Hope is so central to human undertakings that it is likely little would get launched without it. As far back as the first century CE, the Roman philosopher Pliny the Elder said, "Hope is the pillar that holds up the world." Hope, according to Anthony Reading, professor and author, is an "anticipatory emotion," always oriented to the future.[2] Our belief that we possess the ability to bring our hopes into being involves faith. We define faith as the capacity to hold on to ideas, beliefs, or possibilities in the absence of tangible evidence to support them. Ultimately, the voluntary decision to act is taken when our hope drives us to trust that our faith will be rewarded with a better future than what we are experiencing in the present. That, in a nutshell, is the mental basis for optimism.

In chapter 2, we described the brain as the organ that permits our mind to travel through time. We are the only creatures that are able to separate ourselves from our immediate circumstances and travel with our mind's eye to an infinite number of imagined futures. We are also the only creatures that are spurred into action in the present moment in pursuit of that imagined future. Optimism tickles us with desire. The brain's pleasure centers provide electrical and chemical enthusiasm to the higher brain centers so they spur us to act on our hopes and dreams. After all, dreams that aren't followed by actions to achieve them are hollow and devoid of true purpose.

Here's a story: A scientist was studying optimism. One subject was a young boy who maintained a sunny, optimistic outlook under any conceivable condition. To find the limits of the boy's optimism, the scientist filled a windowless room with horse dung. He then sent the boy into the room. Later the scientist opened the door, expecting to discover the boy overcome with sadness about the realities of his foul environment. Instead, he found that the boy had disappeared. Shocked—there were no exits from the room—he called out for the boy. He heard a faint voice saying, "Over here!" The scientist discovered that the boy had dug a tunnel deep into the pile of dung. When the scientist asked him what he was doing, the boy cheerfully called back, "With this much poop around, there has to be a pony in here somewhere!"

The story brings a smile to most people's faces, but it also touches on this chapter's main theme. Optimism is not an unchangeable trait or characteristic that is hardwired into us, like the color of our eyes. *Optimism is actually a skill.* As with all skills, some of us show more basic talent for it than others, but almost all of us can improve our level of optimism with practice.

Can We Have Too Much of a Good Thing?

Optimism makes us like a tightrope walker. On one side of the taut wire is despair. Without enough optimism, we lose hope, give up, and become unable to connect to the joy in life. Martin Seligman, renowned psychologist, researcher, and author, called this phenomenon "learned helplessness," which is essentially an acquired belief based on real-life experiences that tells us we can't escape from a negative situation, no matter what we do.[3] When helpless, we remain convinced our dilemma is inescapable, even when faced with concrete options to escape. Our own negative perceptions create a self-imposed mental prison.

On the other side of the tightrope wire is the world of Pollyanna. When leaning too far in her direction, we let unbridled optimism become so divorced from what is actually achievable that it grows into fantasy-filled delusion. This form of delusion is not limited to individuals with mental illness; it can show up in anyone who is immune to the influence of facts. To walk the wire between these two poles of experience, we must balance far-reaching aspiration with practical grounding in the real world.

Understanding optimism's life-enhancing benefits motivates us to seek ways to increase optimism and obtain the elusive benefits, like joy, that it can confer.

A Spoonful of Optimism
Helps the Setbacks Go Down

At its evolutionary core, optimism is a brain-based coping strategy that helped our early ancestors to survive when the odds of survival were often stacked against them. Optimism isn't the only survival strategy, and it is not always the best strategy, but it clearly has its benefits. It is said that good things come to those who wait. The saying implies that when a reward isn't immediately available, optimism helps motivate us to remain patient while seeking paths to obtain the reward. Abraham Lincoln revised that idea, saying, "Things may come to those who wait, but only the things left by those who hustle." While these sayings seem to emphasize entirely different behaviors—patience versus hustling—they share the idea of *persistence*. Both involve the ability to hang in there, staying the course by either passively but patiently waiting for the anticipated reward or actively chasing after it.

Research shows that high dopamine levels help maintain a persistent focus on the anticipated reward.[4] Dopamine is our attention molecule (see chapters 2 and 3). People with higher levels of dopamine not only are rated as more optimistic, but they stay focused and anticipate higher levels of pleasure with a reward they persistently and optimistically pursue.[5] In a world where the odds of success or even survival were low, optimism grew out of the ability

- to imagine a future goal,
- to ignore or downplay the long odds of achieving it,
- to show persistence by stubborn patience or focused hustle, and
- to *overestimate* the pleasure of the reward that is the object or goal of the pursuit.

These characteristics stacked the survival odds in our ancestors' favor. These optimism building blocks are essential to getting back up, dusting ourselves off, and getting back on the proverbial horse. Life guarantees that we will suffer setbacks and outright defeat at some points. Optimism assures that we don't give up. It assists us to learn something positive and useful from our negative experiences.[6]

Our Positivity Bias

Although writers have emphasized that we are born with a negativity bias that orients us toward fear, risk avoidance, and pessimism,[7] there is also good evidence that we counterbalance this tendency through a positivity bias. Our brains are divided into two halves (the left and right hemispheres). Each contributes a unique ingredient to balanced optimism.

We function best when there is a healthy balance between the left and right's particular orientations. The right hemisphere sees the world from a big-picture point of view that is closely tied to immediate experience. It is also associated with more sober emotions, a pessimistic outlook that can reduce unhealthy and careless risk taking. The left hemisphere, on the other hand, is associated with positive emotions and an optimistic outlook that is grounded in past experience. When a person's left hemisphere is underactive or their right hemisphere is overactive, the person tends to express a depressed outlook. A balanced brain serves as a buffer against depression. Optimism and pessimism exist on a biological and emotional continuum that reflects the relative contributions of each brain hemisphere.

As we age, the bumps and bruises of life accumulate. Aging can increase the risk of becoming worn down, feeling defeated, becoming embittered, and giving up.[8] The high rates of depression in older age reinforce this concern. However, aging research shows a silver lining that should not be underestimated. Healthy aging is associated with an *increase* in optimism.[9]

We can learn diverse lessons from any given experience. Older adults with high levels of optimism tend to show a mild mental blindness for negative aspects of an experience. They put a positive spin on experience, even if that reflects a slight distortion of the facts. Their optimism reflects a subtle but healthy delusion that lowers the sting of the negative and increases the focus on the positive aspects of an experience.

Higher levels of optimism across adulthood are associated with a veritable wish list of health benefits. A study of more than 150,000 adults from 142 countries conducted in 2013[10] showed that people with more optimistic outlooks had

- stronger and healthier hearts,
- lower levels of "bad" cholesterol,
- better ability to handle life stressors,
- greater immune system functioning,
- reduced risk of strokes,
- increased ability to regulate their emotions effectively, and
- longer lifespans!

One of the most interesting findings from this type of research reveals that optimistic older adults aren't simply more likely to wear rose-colored glasses. They actually show thicker, denser neurons in the brain area associated with evaluating emotional aspects of the social environment (the anterior cingulate cortex and the amygdala).[11] As we have seen, our brain is trainable. Practicing optimism changes the brain. Using the mind to engage in brain-changing practices confers important health benefits that make living a long life that much more pleasurable and fulfilling.

Teflon-Coating the Mind

If the first half of your life was relatively challenge-free, you might be optimistic that the second half of your life would involve more of the same. You could be right, but only in a most fragile and superficial manner. Research suggests that being born with a silver spoon in one's mouth isn't associated with long-term optimism. A privileged early life can actually result in a more difficult time adjusting to adversity encountered later in life. If early needs and wants have been too easily satisfied, you may miss out on one of the most important sources of optimism.

For optimism to be useful, it must be *hardy*. If optimism bursts like a fragile balloon the moment it is pricked by life's adversity, what good is it? Optimism becomes a hardy and resilient part of a person's outlook when it has been field-tested over and over. Out of encounters with life's darker experiences can emerge the kind of deeply rooted optimism that stubbornly persists despite all manner of challenges. When properly exercised, optimism functions like a Teflon coating that sloughs off the bumps and bruises faced in older life.

While optimism is rooted in our biology, it is expressed in daily life through our psychology and behavior. Our mind holds the key to growing *resilient* optimism by orchestrating the brain's activities. The mind is the bridge between possibility and actuality. When the mind is optimistic:

- The brain does not encode into memory mildly or moderately negative experiences as strongly, so one is more likely to persist when first encountering frustrations.
- The posterior parietal cortex (PPC) of the brain talks more actively with the frontal cortex and the brain's motivation centers to set up action plans for pursuing long-term goals with vigor and determination.

- The brain is better able to pay *selective* attention to what is most likely to lead to achieving the goal, and tune out the rest.

- You *perceive* that the circumstances of your daily world are less random and more influenced by your actions than they really are. That makes you less subject to fear.

- You perceive yourself to have greater self-efficacy, which is the belief that you have the necessary resources *within you* to achieve what you set out to achieve.

- The brain supports more positive self-esteem and reduces the risk of depression, which are key ingredients for long-term happiness and contentment.

- The forces of neuroplasticity rewire the brain's neural circuits so that optimism becomes a *default* outlook, occurring more automatically.

This does not mean that all fear, pain, loss, or suffering must be forever banished from life. Paradoxically, optimism is a highly refined *realism*. Optimism emerges from the actual details and challenges of life, but it does not allow us to be defined by or limited to those details. Optimism acknowledges that suffering is simply and unavoidably part of life's journey, but at the same time, it reminds us that contentment, joy, and happiness can nevertheless be attained with persistent and determined effort.

Optimism Filters

No matter where on the optimism-pessimism continuum you find yourself, developing resilient and balanced optimism rests on three information-processing filters. Think of them as lenses through which information about you and your world are actively filtered.

All three mental filters have their roots in the biology of our brain. In particular, a small area called the inferior frontal gyrus (IFG) on the left and right sides of the brain is selectively activated depending upon whether a person maintains an optimistic or pessimistic perception of their environment.[12] The left IFG is especially good at generating and maintaining positive emotional states. A sunny disposition and positive outlook depend on left IFG activation. The right IFG excels at detecting change and adjusting emotional states, especially anxiety and fear. The right IFG also sounds a pessimistic warning in response to changes in environmental circumstances that potentially pose a threat.[13] Each individual balances the left and right IFG in ways unique to their personality style. This balance is a starting point. It is not fixed. It does not define or determine the potential for change and growth in optimism that can occur. From that starting point there is the potential for growing your optimism level through the practices we outline below.

Filter One: The Selection Filter

The first optimism-building filter involves selective attention. We can't be everywhere at once. Without paying attention to where we *choose* to be, we will find ourselves wherever our habits take us, including the habit of seeing the world as a half-empty glass. On which aspects of your experience do you dwell? What is your default selective attention filter?

Learning to use the selective attention filter helps people to notice aspects of their inner and outer experience that have existed all along but were until now overlooked. For example, our brain processes a tremendous amount of bodily activity that never reaches conscious awareness, such as microadjustments in our heart rate and blood pressure. Some aspects of unconscious brain activity can be brought to conscious awareness with practice. This is where we enter the world of selective attention. These patterns of noticing, feeling, thinking, and reacting form the basis of what we call our *personality*. Personality is nothing more than the repeated patterns of living that characterize who we are from our most basic physiological level to our most abstract, higher-level thinking. Through the use of selective attention, we can create new patterns of noticing to replace old patterns that sustained fear or other forms of unhappiness. Repeated patterns persist as habits so long as they are not brought to awareness, examined, and modified. In other words, this filter allows us to make active *choices* about how we perceive ourselves and our social world.

How do you learn to actively choose your perceptual reality so that optimism can grow? Imagine you are a wedding photographer. You are in a reception room where the couple is greeting guests. If you focus your camera lens only on the groom's parents—an odd choice perhaps, but still possible—the essential interactions of the couple with their friends and family will be missed. If you miss photographing the new couple, you will not last long as a wedding photographer. A good wedding photographer is able to shift the focus of the camera's lens from the couple to friends, to family, to wedding cake, to table settings, to the dance floor, and back to the couple so that the images capture the unique feel of the event. The photographer actively and with conscious deliberation *selects* the focus that is most appropriate to each unfolding moment. As the photographer gains experience, the conscious effort needed to selectively capture the right wedding shot becomes more automatic because the perceptual habits born of repeated practice become more deeply engrained. The photographer's practice may thrive as a result.

Since what you attend to largely determines what you see, the focus of your selective attention creates a "glass half-full" or "glass half-empty" view. Studies from neuropsychology, for example, have clearly shown that the eyes of people with depression focus on features of photographs that reflect sadness, danger, or other negative elements. The eyes of subjects without depression zeroed in on photographic features that reflected joy, contentment, or other positive emotions.[14]

To grow optimism, you must actively and mindfully *select* the focus of your attention. Notice what features of your inner or outer environment you are drawn to pay attention to and whether those features are helpful. Do those features help you to more deeply engage with others or to withdraw and detach from them? Optimism grows in an atmosphere of deeper connection with others.

Filter Two: The Address of Control

The second feature involved in growing optimism is the perceptual address at which your sense of control resides. This psychological address is called locus of control (LoC). People with an *internal* LoC perceive that they are in a prime position to influence what happens in their daily lives. They perceive that it is their actions and their decisions that primarily influence what happens to them. As a result, people with an internal LoC tend to be proactive in how they approach concerns or how they go about achieving goals they have set. They deeply believe that their actions matter.

On the other end of the LoC continuum are people with an *external* locus of control. They perceive their world as subject to the influence of external forces. The boss's decision matters more than their own actions. The weather dictates how their day will go. Their genetics trump the influence of their self-care practices. Their future health therefore becomes a function of many factors over which they perceive little influence or control. As a result of this psychological lens, external LoC-based individuals tend to be more passive about their daily choices. Why not? Their perceptual lens tells them that their actions don't really matter all that much. Therefore, it makes more sense not to waste the time and energy tilting at windmills.

But locus of control *does* matter. When your LoC resides deep within yourself, you're more comfortable taking calculated risks to make changes in your life. Not only do your actions matter, but you matter as a person. You know that one individual *can* make a difference. Operating from such a position, you may be more compelled to take on projects that make tangible differences in other people's lives.

A physician friend has been traveling to Haiti several times each year to work in a makeshift hospital on that impoverished island nation. He tends to the needs of people coming to the hospital with all manner of ailments that would be treated quite routinely if such people were seen in a US emergency room. In the years he has been going there, little has changed in the country as a whole. The conditions remain appallingly backward and people die "for no reason at all" except that they happened to be born to a life in Haiti versus Hawaii. And yet, he travels there every few months, doing what he can for as long as he can, making a difference in the lives of people he doesn't know and won't see again, simply because he knows he can and that his choices matter. That is internalized locus of control in action.

Where is your LoC? Do your actions matter? Can your actions make a small but positive difference in someone else's life today? Can that action orientation become a daily practice for you?

Filter Three: Cause and Effect

When important events happen, we automatically work to make sense of them, to attribute them to a cause. The ability to explain to ourselves the cause of events is fundamental to how our brain and mind operate. We can't stand not knowing. As we age, maintaining a sense of control and influence is a key to sustaining optimism in our lives. The way you make sense of what has happened in your life defines your attributional style. Three dimensions determine attributional style:

- internal-external
- stable-unstable
- global-local

We've already discussed the first of these styles: internal-external. Locus of control determines whether we perceive the cause of an outcome to have come from our own actions or from external factors. For example, "My decision to exercise by walking each day helped me avoid the flu when many other people around me got sick," reflects one who sees the cause as coming from within.

The *stable-unstable* dimension determines whether the cause is viewed as a onetime event or an ongoing influence. A person who says, "I know I won't develop dementia because my whole life I've been able to beat the odds," is showing an internal locus (*I know I can*) and is attributing that internal control to a *stable*, personal quality (*I've* always *been able to . . .*).

The *local-global* variable reflects whether the fall on the ice happened because "I didn't watch where I was going yesterday" (local—a single, identifiable cause unlikely to persist) or whether "I am such a klutz that it is a continuous miracle that I can *ever* get through a day without hurting myself" (global—an ever-present and inescapable cause).

Ascribing outcomes to local events can make them time-limited. This is especially helpful when a negative result is achieved. A local attribution leads you to say, "I can do better next time because there were some unique factors that applied here that are unlikely to reoccur in the future." Attributing outcomes to global factors, on the other hand, especially when they are *personal* and *stable*, can suck the life out of any effort to grow optimism. This is precisely what occurs with individuals who suffer from depression and who exhibit a pessimistic outlook on their future. Their outlook is colored by the belief that when something goes wrong in their lives, it is almost certainly their fault at some level and that this is unlikely to change in the future (it is a *personal* and *stable* attribute).

The awareness of attributional style has helped us better understand depression, a major threat to older individuals. For example, studies of individuals with depression tend to show an overreliance on the three Ps.[15] Negative events are viewed as being *pervasive*. If something bad happened somewhere, the belief is that badness will happen everywhere. In addition, events are invested with *permanence*. If something bad happens now, it is likely to keep on happening. Finally, if something bad happens, it is perceived as having to do with something for which the individual is *personally* responsible (as in *It's all my fault!*).

Pervasive, permanent, and personal: the infamous three Ps. Even in small doses you will feel their influence, whether or not you have depression. In combination, they are a potent recipe for feeling loss of control over your life, and they deal a body blow to efforts at building optimism.

Michael Yapko is a world-renowned expert on how to successfully treat depression and cultivate balanced optimism. What follows are his top eight mental practices for countering depression while also supporting healthy optimism.[16] How many do you regularly practice?

- Balance awareness of your own internal sensations, thoughts, and feelings with a sense of connection to others' thoughts and feelings.
- Watch your tendency to minimize the negative while maximizing the positive (creating risky self-deception).
- Watch your tendency to minimize the positive while maximizing the negative (creating despair and a sense of futility about the future).
- Catch and correct any tendency to perceive that in encounters with others you represent less than half of the overall relationship equation.

- Keep in check tendencies toward perfectionism: when a person is focused on being perfect, the future becomes nothing but a constant threat of failure to be perfect.
- Minimize overgeneralizing to limit the tendency to turn negative molehills into insurmountable mountains.
- Balance how you solicit support from others with the blessing of offering others support.
- Remember to seek alternative viewpoints; no one has a lock on the one and only truth about your future.

The Road to the Land of Optimism

As you go about creating optimism practices that are just right for you, bear in mind what a friend of mine once said: "You exist. You matter. You make sense." What he highlighted are three mind-based affirmations that are a foundation upon which to grow your optimism.

- You exist. You have a physical existence in the world. So long as you draw a breath, your presence in the world is not a fiction or fantasy. Recognizing this inescapable truth helps promote greater appreciation for how you choose to *be present* in the world.
- You matter. Your presence in the world matters. There has never been anyone exactly like you, nor will there ever be another person exactly like you ever again. Your uniqueness is a precious gift. The only thing you can ever be is a fulfillment of the promise of who you already are. In that way, your presence *in* the world can make a meaningful difference *to* the world, especially to that small part of the world that you occupy along with your closest friends and loved ones.

- You make sense. Your life in this world makes sense. Every life has a purpose, a destiny aided by the cultivation of optimism.

Some see the purpose of one's life as predetermined or preordained. The ancient Greeks, for example, talked of fate and destiny as two different forms of the flow of one's life. *Fate* reflects the predetermined direction that your life is believed to follow based on unseen forces that control the universe and, by extension, control you. This is not what we mean when we say every life makes sense. This would mean that what you select to focus on wouldn't ultimately matter because your locus of control would be external. It would be in the hands of the Greeks' menagerie of fickle gods—global, stable, and external.

Living a life that makes unique sense is, in our view, more similar to *destiny*. Through the choices you make, guided by conscious awareness and intentional, thoughtful actions, you gradually work out the basic purpose of your life in a way that brings meaning—sense—to your life. Knowing that your destiny rests in large measure with the choices you make is essential to cultivating resilient optimism. Optimism allows the investment of trust, hope, and strong belief into your choices. Optimism also provides the emotional tenacity necessary to persist with your choices even in the face of adversity. In short, optimism provides the means to achieve your *destiny*, which we define as a life characterized by expression of your inner resources to their highest potential.

Anticipation

Optimism is mental foreplay. Anticipation of a positive outcome in the future gets us excited, aroused, and motivated in the present moment. People who are habitual procrastinators report that the pressure of an impending deadline and the fear of embarrassment or other consequences of missing the deadline finally prompt them to act. Optimists, on the other hand, are motivated less by fear and more by the pleasure they anticipate when they imagine how the future will turn out. Singer-songwriter Carly Simon's "Anticipation" includes the lyrics, "We can never know about the days to come, but we think about them anyway." Therein lies one of the keys for developing resilient optimism. We anticipate the good—and act to bring the good into being!

Robert Sapolsky, a neuroendocrinologist at Stanford University and recipient of the MacArthur Fellowship genius grant, has studied the role of anticipation in goal-directed behavior. Dopamine, the brain's focusing molecule, is released when the situation promising the *possibility* of reward is encountered.[17,18] In the lecture Sapolsky delivered February 15, 2011, to the California Academy of Sciences,[19] he made a point central to consolidating our understanding of the role of optimism in life. What makes human beings unique is the length of time over which we are able to sustain dopamine release in anticipation of the promise of pleasure. With our unique prefrontal brain regions that allow us to mentally travel across time, human beings can anticipate rewards that may not occur for decades.

In fact, says Sapolsky, we humans possess the unparalleled ability to organize our lives toward events we believe won't even occur in our lifetimes! Examples include the anticipation of a reward that will come after death (for instance, heaven) or the willingness to sacrifice over the course of a lifetime to provide a better life for our children or to leave the world a better place for the next generation. To stubbornly and single-mindedly pursue goals that we believe we will never directly benefit from is perhaps the most powerful example of the capacity of optimism to determine the course of our lives.

Marinate in the Good

Optimism represents the third leg (along with flexibility and curiosity) of the three-legged stool characterizing the role of the mind for aging well. The capacity to be optimistic is wired deeply into our brain. So is the capacity for pessimism. Optimism and pessimism represent two ends of a continuum, forever shifting according to the fortunes and dictates of our daily lives. The role of the *mind* is to gradually shift the fulcrum between optimism and pessimism so that we become more inclined to lean toward an optimistic perspective on life.

Those living into their eighties often say that aging isn't for the faint-hearted. Aging is a daily challenge. No one reaches that stage of life without scars. The miracle is how few abandon their hope that in spite of their travails, good things can still lie ahead. Anne Frank wrote, "It's really a wonder that I haven't dropped all my ideals, because they seem so absurd and impossible to carry out. Yet I keep them, because in spite of everything I still believe that people are really good at heart." What are your central ideals? What are the core beliefs that guide your decision making and reflect your attitudes about how you will imbue your life with meaning and purpose? How do you assure that your life matters and makes sense?

Since life is so full of challenges and obstacles, Anne Frank again has something important to teach us. She wrote, "And finally I twist my heart round again, so that the bad is on the outside and the good is on the inside, and keep on trying to find a way of becoming what I would so like to be, and could be, if there weren't any other people living in the world." She was describing what we call marinating in the good. Actively maintain a positive focus about the future largely irrespective of what others think or say. Deliberately seek to visualize positive possibilities of future outcomes. Anticipate the positive reward you can achieve through your persistent efforts. Like the little engine that could, rehearse the mantra "I think I can. I think I can. I think I can." Each time these practices are engaged, your mind is incrementally rewiring your brain to grow optimism. And like Anne Frank, you become more and more capable of being the person you would "so like to be" while relying on your personal resources to manifest your highest and best self.

◇◇

A Helpful Practice for Growing Optimism through Positive Selective Attention

Learning to express your highest self begins with optimism that you *can* manifest that higher self. Developing such optimism requires a long view that leapfrogs over current challenges. Fear and worry, on the other hand, foster a nearsighted outlook. Selective attention, when combined with mindful awareness practices, allows us to acknowledge obstacles without being sidetracked or derailed by them. It is an important building block to optimism. Here is a simple exercise for building mindful selective attention skills.

Commit to devoting ten to twenty minutes per day to gradually developing your selective attention abilities. Establish a set place (and a set time) to practice. Sit in a chair that supports your back while your feet can be firmly on the floor. Place your hands gently in your lap. Breathe in. Feel the air filling your lungs as though it were water being poured into a large pitcher. Then, when filled, hold the air in your lungs for a few moments before slowly "pouring" the air out with a gentle and controlled exhale. Repeat this several times. You may find it more comfortable to allow your eyes to close on one of the exhales. Notice also that with each exhale there is a natural release of muscle tension from the body and a momentary release of the intensity of any thoughts and a softening of any emotions you are feeling.

Over the next few minutes, direct your attention to the following four steps. Focus your attention on one of the four steps for each complete cycle of breathing in, momentarily holding the air in your lungs, and then slowly releasing it with your exhale. Then focus your attention on the next step. When you have completed the four steps with four cycles of breath, start over with the first step. Keep following this sequence for ten minutes. With practice, increase the time you practice to twenty minutes.

Here are the four steps.

1. As you breathe in and then out, notice what you feel in your physical body. You may notice areas of comfort and discomfort. You may notice areas that are warmer or cooler. You may notice the feel of air on your skin or the gentle pulse of your heart's beat in the tip of a finger. Just focus on what you feel during this breath.

2. As you breathe in and then out, notice what you sense in the room around you. You may open your eyes or choose for them to remain closed. Notice what you hear or what you smell or, if your eyes are open, what your eyes take in. Just notice what surrounds you during this breath.

3. As you breathe in and then out, allow yourself to consider how nothing is permanent. Everything changes. The breath comes in and the breath goes out. The heart beats and the heart relaxes. Thoughts rise up and subside to be replaced by new thoughts. Even feelings and sensations rise up, shift, and become something new. Everything is renewed in each moment. Focus on this idea during this cycle of breath.

4. As you breathe in and then out, notice how you can allow what is happening inside or outside you and around you—in your body, in your mind, and in the space around your body—to come and go without needing to grab on to it. Practice simply observing what comes and goes without getting attached to it. Things come, things go, and you are still here, more and more able to selectively choose what with growing optimism you want to pursue—the kind of future you are capable of creating. Focus on this during this cycle of breath. Return to step one and repeat.

Part 4

The Voyage Home

Journeying toward an Awakened Heart

We are not provided with wisdom, we must discover it for ourselves,
after a journey through the wilderness which no one else can take for us,
and effort which no one can spare us.

—MARCEL PROUST

Homer's *Odyssey*, written nearly three thousand years ago, is one of literature's most enduring stories about the inevitability of encountering obstacle after obstacle as important personal goals are pursued. As we have attempted to show, the journey along life's path is less about avoiding obstacles than it is about making important choices about how to face them.

We have highlighted two sets of practices to support both a youthful brain (nutrition, sleep, and exercise) and a vibrant mind (curiosity, flexibility, and optimism). In this final section, we consider three additional steps you can take toward a wise heart. We will focus on what gives life its meaning and purpose—our capacity for empathy, the quality of our connections with others, and the promise of being authentically ourselves.

As with Odysseus, the legacy of our lives is defined by how we find our way home to ourselves and, in turn, how that self functions in the world. The choices and actions we take determine whether we ultimately live an authentic life that acknowledges the gift of our uniqueness, and whether we use that gift to positively impact the world we all share.

10

A Youthful Brain Is Empathic

Key 7

Empathy is about finding echoes of another person in yourself.
—MOHSIN HAMID

Key Concepts

- Empathy arises from brain regions that regulate the quality of our relationships to others.
- Practicing empathy skills improves the ability to regulate your mind and behavior.
- Empathy is *interactive*; it influences the brains of those with whom you interact.
- When empathy is actively practiced, calmness, contentment, and satisfaction can flourish.
- Developing empathic children may be the greatest legacy we can transmit to the next generation.

AGNES: Empathy Instructor Extraordinaire

The Massachusetts Institute of Technology (MIT) may seem a strange place to begin a discussion about the role of empathy in successful aging.

But in fact, researchers at MIT studied the capacity to put ourselves into someone else's felt experience, which is thought by many to be among the highest of human achievements. Everything from avoidance of war to the establishment of lifelong loving relationships depends, in some measure, on the ability to appreciate the other's perspective, to feel their feelings, and to be able to "walk a mile in their shoes." And to this end, a product designed at MIT seeks to open a window into empathy, aging, and the creation of a more aging-sensitive world.

Joseph Coughlin, a professor at MIT, recognized that our culture is physically designed in ways oblivious to the comfort and accessibility needs of older adults. Beginning in 1999, his lab developed AGNES (Age Gain Now Empathy System).[1] It is a suit containing weights, specialized clothing and shoes, elastic straps, colored goggles, and other headgear carefully designed to force the wearer to mimic the experience of moving about in the world as an older adult. Research volunteers wear the suit while walking, climbing stairs, shopping, or otherwise engaging in the routine activities of daily living. They quickly discover how little of our cultural landscape is designed with the elderly in mind. Fatigue rapidly sets in. Frustration levels rise. Removing a gallon-sized jug of juice from a grocery store's upper shelf suddenly becomes an effortful labor. The experience quickly creates feelings of empathy in the volunteers for what it is like for older adults to simply move about their world on a day-to-day basis.

The results of AGNES suit studies have been used by some of the largest and most recognizable US companies to redesign their products to better attend to the needs of our graying society. AGNES influenced the product design process of huge corporations by having researchers literally walk a mile in the shoes of older adults.

The power and influence of empathic experience should not be underestimated. Jack Handey, an American humorist, agrees: "Before criticizing someone, walk a mile in their shoes. Then when you do criticize them, you will be a mile away and have their shoes!" Funny, but his line also captures the idea that where empathy operates, criticism fades. Empathy draws us closer to one another, while criticism spawns defensiveness and interpersonal distance.

As we hope to make clear in this chapter, developing and maintaining high levels of empathy become especially important as we age. Studies show that empathy declines with aging unless it is deliberately and regularly cultivated.[2] Therefore, a major method of staving off feelings of disconnection or social isolation following loss is to actively exercise empathy skills throughout one's life. In fact, updated studies of older adults show that declines in empathy have less to do with an aging brain than with how that person exercised their empathy-building skills earlier in life.[3]

Discovering the Roots of Empathy

Honeybees don't need empathy. They pollinate the flowers and fruits of the world just fine without it. Swans don't require empathy either. Their grace and beauty shine brightly without the benefit of empathic skills. Most creatures live in a world of simple action and reaction. People, on the other hand—and most mammals—occupy a different and more complex world. Empathy is vital to successfully negotiating their way through the complex maze of social group relationships.

The *insula* is a structure that sits deep within the brain, where it is richly linked to other brain areas that process sensations (hypothalamus) within the body and basic emotions (amygdala) that are aroused from situations outside the body. Occupying the pickle-in-the-middle position, the insula links together raw feelings with the particular state of the body that is connected to those feelings. The relevance of this nerve pathway with regard to empathy became clearer through studies done early in the last century by William James and Carl Lange.[4]

Their experiments showed that when there is a threat, the body is first alerted that danger looms, and *only then* does the threat reach conscious awareness. So we experience emotions in response to sensations aroused in our bodies, not the other way around! In other words, we *know* about our feelings *through* our bodies (embodied awareness).

About twenty years ago, scientists studying the motor region (the area responsible for goal-directed actions) of monkey brains made a startling discovery. The brains of the monkeys *fired* when they observed researchers engaged in activities like reaching for a tool or piece of food. More important, the researchers found that even though the monkeys were merely *watching,* the very same areas were activated in their brains as those activated in the researchers' own brains by reaching for the food. Having monkeys reach for food wasn't the important discovery here. It was the discovery that monkeys learned about how to obtain food by a method they wouldn't normally use because their brain activity mimicked the brains of the researchers actually doing the eating. This was a real, live version of "monkey see, monkey do." One brain's activation pattern was imprinted into the brain activation pattern of the observer monkey, making it much easier for the observer monkey to learn the new behavior quickly. The monkeys showed they could learn complex social actions by mimicking what the researchers did.[5,6] The name given to those nerve cells that fire while mimicking the purposeful behavior of others is *mirror neurons.*

Many years and countless experiments later, a blueprint emerged for constructing the human capacity for empathy: When we observe someone doing something that is important to us, our mirror neurons fire off in our own brain. The firing pattern in our brain allows us to mimic and mentally reproduce what we see the other person do, as well as the emotions associated with what they are doing. Mirror neurons, with the support of other key brain structures, help us to generate an internal map in our brain of the pattern of electrical signals that are firing in the brain of the *other* person. In that way, we are able to read, with remarkable accuracy, the feeling state that the other person is experiencing!

The mirror neurons create a highly sophisticated speed-reading system. In milliseconds we can read whether a person's smile is sincere; the mimicking capabilities of the mirror neuron systems allow us to read the feeling state of the smiling person, which quickly helps us intuitively sense whether to deepen our connection to that person or to pull back. This is empathy: the ability to feel the feeling that the other person is feeling as the person is experiencing it. Empathy creates an emotional echo that reverberates within us. The first echoes of this reverberation are formed by the patterns of connection to our caregivers very early in life.

Right World, Left World

At birth we are entirely dependent for our survival on those who care for us. We require a multilayered connection to others in order to live and grow. Attachment research has identified the profound impact that the quality of the early caregiving connection has on us over the course of our lives.[7] This interpersonal parent-child connection constitutes a multilane, emotional superhighway. The traffic on this highway flows in both directions: caregiver to infant and back again. The quality of the interaction with caregivers etches complex patterns into the infant's developing brain that regulate arousal, reward, safety, excitement, and danger. These form the foundations for empathy.

At first, the attentive caregiver *reads* our emotional and physical needs and responds to them. After years of being read by others, we gradually learn to read those needs within ourselves. Later, having learned to read ourselves, we become capable of reading others. This cycle of being read, reading ourselves, and later reading others binds us to one another in endless loops of empathy-based social connections. From infancy through the early years of childhood, increasingly complex interaction patterns are absorbed, shaping the young person's ability to regulate his/her own behavior in an expanding range of interpersonal encounters. That is why these early patterns of interacting can so powerfully shape the kind and quality of your relationships throughout life.

Alan Schore[8,9,10] is one of the major figures to clarify the nature of the reciprocal relationship between brains as people interact with one another.[11,12,13] Much of his research looks at the special role played by the *right* brain hemisphere in human relationships. The right hemisphere is better able than the left to perceive what is new as a relationship unfolds moment by moment. The right hemisphere is more strongly connected to the body, enabling you to sense the physical and sensory impact of interactions with others. The right hemisphere perceives the nonverbal aspects of our interactions, like the subtle facial expressions which make up 50 to 90 percent of what gets communicated during an encounter. Nonverbal signals provide the emotional context for interpreting the words being spoken. The right hemisphere of the brain is fundamentally the relationship hemisphere, whereas the left hemisphere is the storekeeper of the memories of those experiences.

Intimate Aging

When people gather to celebrate life's events—anniversaries of births, marriages, deaths, sobriety dates, holidays, retirements, or perhaps first dates—they invariably reminisce about the past. They catch up with each other by filling in the blanks of what has occurred since the last time they were in contact with each other. Thinking back to recall earlier shared experiences brings people together and fosters nostalgia and closeness. Emotional intimacy takes that closeness a step or two farther. Emotional intimacy is a bonding agent that keeps relationships alive, vibrant, and loving. Of course people vary in their ability to develop intimacy,[14] but regardless of where you are on that continuum, you can grow in your human capacity for greater intimacy.

Maintaining and even deepening intimacy in the second half of life is important for several reasons. Aging is filled with pervasive stresses that intensify over time. People who are more intimately wired to others tend to withstand the impact of stress with greater hardiness and may even thrive. An intimate connection to a partner or a network of friends generates a protective buffer that dampens the impact of losses and setbacks that accumulate over time.

The capacity for intimacy is inextricably linked to the capacity for empathy.[15] Both are rooted in our neurobiology. Both are capable of expanding and rewiring the brain to create a lasting source of closeness and comfort. Marsha Lucas has nicely captured seven characteristics exhibited by people in healthy relationships.[16] Notice how many of the characteristics paraphrased here involve the set of skills we have promoted for preserving a youthful brain.

- Learn how to regulate or manage your body's reactions to stressors.
- Develop the ability to modulate your response to fear.
- Cultivate skills that build emotional resiliency.
- Grow your capacity to respond to challenges in a flexible manner.
- Develop insight that leads to knowing yourself more honestly.
- Learn to tune in to your own feelings and those of others (empathy).
- Shift your outlook from "me" to "we."

Practicing these seven skills can make genuine intimacy more accessible. It is the quality of the encounter between two people that comes to define the nature of the relationship. The goal of intimacy is to recognize and honor what is unique and whole about the other.

Aging with Empathy

Empathy's role in staying on the path to joy varies as it sometimes supports the growth of joy and sometimes challenges it, especially as we age. Nature seems to have anticipated that. For example, adults entering their sixties showed greater ability to empathize with people facing unfortunate circumstances. They also showed greater ability to see the good in difficult circumstances when compared to people in their twenties or forties, according to research conducted by R. Levenson and others. [17,18]

The research also suggests that there is a major shift in the second half of life toward establishing close interpersonal relationships. For example, Gisela Labouvie-Vief has found evidence that older adults enter a formal stage of cognitive development that supports long-term commitment and that includes a stronger ability to integrate emotion and logical thinking when making complex decisions. While this capacity makes its initial appearance in early adulthood, her research suggests it continues to mature and strengthen, meaning that in the second half of life, the commitments into which adults can enter are potentially richer and more complex.[19] Nevertheless, the strong capacity for empathy seen in older adults is a powerful foundation upon which compassion for self and others can grow, and current research hails the role of such compassion skills in sustaining and building resilient health skills well into older age.[20]

Depth of connection becomes more important than the number of people with whom to connect. Ironically, the emphasis on relationship closeness exposes older adults to more encounters with sadness. Today's older adults live much longer than in the past. But in our society, those extra years are often spent at greater geographic distance from children and extended family. Exposure to physical illness and the decline and death of loved ones are additional sources of sadness. And a society too often fixated on youth and beauty becomes yet another source of sadness by conveying a message that loss of youth means loss of value or worth.

In light of these experiences, maintaining empathy as we age is important both for the individual and for society. For example, individuals high in empathy skills have healthier hearts. They also tend to be more open-hearted, showing higher levels of compassion and expressed concern toward others. Since empathy involves tuning into one's self and then using that inner knowledge to become attuned to others, empathy also becomes important for building more connected social communities in which people in the second half of their lives play vital roles. When sympathy abounds, positive social benefits begin to blossom. Studies have shown relationships between higher empathy skills and altruism,[21] with a range of successful business-savvy practices having clear economic benefits for others,[22] and with more modest, simple actions that make random encounters between strangers more pleasant.[23]

More Important Than Bedtime Stories

Storytelling is an important practice for exercising empathy. Author Paul John Eakin captured this idea when he wrote that "our life stories are not merely *about* us but in an inescapable and profound way *are* us," (emphasis added).[24] Cell biologist and author Bruce Lipton says that our beliefs about relationships, as reflected in our stories, are so powerful that they shape our biology, right down to the level of how genes in our cells are turned on or off.

While stories arise from past experience, they can also modify future experience by refining our recollection of the past, emphasizing greater optimism and a more positive outlook going forward. Since our stories are changeable, the implication is that our biology is changeable too, as shown by research into the neuroplastic potential of the brain.

Increasing empathy in daily life involves several practices that show up over and over in the research literature. They draw upon skills you have already been exposed to, especially the triad of flexibility, curiosity, and optimism described in part 3. Below are practical methods you can use to increase your empathy. Your brain and your social network will thank you.

Practice Active Listening

Active listening is a multilevel form of communicating. By listening *to* the other, you allow yourself to be changed *by* the other. When you listen with your heart (right brain) and not just with your intellect (left brain), you will find yourself drawn into what the other person is *saying* and also into what they are *experiencing* (you will feel empathy). As a result, you will be affected more deeply by their story. That is why active listening rests upon your ability to tolerate vulnerability. Actively listening with vulnerability means to be actively affected by the other's experience in ways that lead to a shift in your understanding of the person's experience. This often leads to greater acceptance of the other's perspective (not necessarily agreeing, but accepting) and an increase in feelings of compassion for that perspective. Guidelines for active listening include

- not interrupting.
- asking questions that invite others to keep expressing what they need or want to express.
- taking care not to give advice or tell them what you think they *should* do or minimize their feelings. Any of these can turn heartfelt empathy into judgmental sympathy or pity.

- reflecting back what you understand them to be saying so they have an opportunity both to feel heard and to restate anything that has been misunderstood.
- through your body language, communicating that you are listening (for example, maintaining eye contact, facing them, leaning in toward them, nodding your head).

Practice Open-Minded Curiosity

Curiosity is the mental attitude that says, "There is something here for me to discover." It is the antithesis of prejudgment, bias, or prejudice. When curious, you are drawn *toward* others to discover through nonjudgmental questions what is interesting, attractive, intriguing, and novel about them. Perhaps most important, a curious mind develops your empathy skills because it assumes the other has something important to offer. To discover what that something is, you will have to persist in your efforts to make that enriching connection. At the end of the day, the empathic connection gets organized around the similarities you share rather than the differences that might divide and separate you.

Practice Transformational Imagination

Empathy felt toward someone creates bonds that can generate synergy, meaning more can be accomplished together than separately. At times, those efforts become powerful agents for social change. Children of Peace, for example, is a nonpartisan organization that brings together Palestinian, Israeli, Turkish, and other Middle Eastern children ages fourteen to seventeen to forge lasting friendships through arts, education, health, and sports programming. Participants transform their dim and prejudiced views of one another into a vision of peaceful coexistence that transcends current regional realities. Another example is the Jay Phillips

Center for Interfaith Learning, which aligns the efforts at three universities to promote greater understanding across people of different faith traditions and unites their efforts toward a greater common social good.

Do Silver Linings Have Dark Clouds?

Clearly, empathy is a good quality, but is it possible to have too much empathy? Indeed, there are risks from unregulated empathy, and the metaphor of a camera's lens helps us understand them. Photographers regulate the intensity of light falling on the camera sensor by varying how widely the lens aperture is open. If the lens is open too wide, it may allow in excessive light and the image can be blown out.

So too with empathy. Chronically keeping the empathy dial on maximum can allow in too much of other people's experiences. Your stress coping system can be overwhelmed by too much vulnerability, or what psychologists call poor interpersonal boundaries. Over time, this can result in a variety of stress-related conditions.

While the benefits of empathy are clear, unregulated empathy can produce the emotional equivalent of a repetitive stress injury. It is often in the second half of life when these mental injuries show up in the form of burnout, including diminished mental performance, physical illnesses, and emotional numbing. People in caregiving positions, like health care workers, teachers, and law enforcement personnel, have the highest rates of burnout. The term for this type of burnout is *vicarious traumatization*. As the name implies, bearing witness to people's suffering can have very negative health consequences. Being overexposed to other people's pain and struggles can exact a negative toll.

Burnout may have a neurobiological basis involving negative neuroplastic change.[25,26] Under the stress of constant input, such as an overempathic connection to others, the hippocampus (the brain area involved in encoding new experience) seems to go dormant. Fewer nerve cells germinate. The sprouting of new brain cells (neurogenesis) declines, leaving one less resilient in the face of future stresses.

The good news is that the risk of overexposure to empathy is quite manageable with active and consistent self-care. This includes play and laughter, along with the core practices of exercise, sleep, and sound nutrition outlined earlier in this book. Also, engaging in the regular practice of healthy empathy tells your brain to secrete more serotonin.[27] When bathed in calm contentment as a result of higher brain serotonin levels, you can deepen your connection to others, and you have a greater desire to do so. The strengthening of your social networks offsets any risk from being more emotionally open and vulnerable in your expression of empathy.[28] Active self-care and rich social networks are our way of adjusting our emotional aperture to avoid feeling blown out or burned out.

The Repair of the World

Empathy is an acquired ability that depends upon the social interactions and environment in which we are raised. Empathy is an *emergent* aspect of being human. In other words, our genetic capacity for empathy is maximized or stifled depending upon how the empathy circuits within the brain are exercised. Those circuits cannot be exercised in isolation. In fact, isolation is quite unhealthy for the development of empathy. Empathy must, as we said earlier, emerge from and get tuned by our early encounters with caregivers. The tuning process later gets refined in the context of our primary adult relationships.

As we have shown, the cultivation of empathy ultimately depends upon the quality of the relationship we have with ourselves. It is difficult to express to others what we don't feel toward ourselves. Even simply being kind to someone else becomes harder when we harbor anger toward ourselves or sling harsh messages at our own hearts over perceived flaws and failures. The paradox is that acting with compassion and empathy toward others becomes much more natural when we express compassion and empathy toward our own inescapable short-comings and imperfections. You don't have to be perfect to be great!

Judaism contains a principle called *tikkun olam*, or *the repair of the world*. The idea is that in the course of our lives, we are all obligated to leave the world better off than it was when we inherited it. There is a spiritual aspect to this principle that involves doing our individual part in restoring the world to a state of divinely inspired perfection. However, nowhere is there the assumption that any one of us alone will succeed in bringing the world to a state of perfection, nor is there an expectation that we will ever achieve that perfect state ourselves. We are and always will remain flawed. Why, then, is the principle of *tikkun olam* so appealing?

Using our lives to make a positive difference in the world—to do our part to repair it—involves both *aspiration* and *legacy*. The principle generates an aspiration to create a future that relies on our being our best selves. The principle involves legacy in that it encourages us to consider what the result of our life's efforts will leave to the generations that follow us. Both topics are especially poignant as we enter the second half of our lives. To practice empathy in our intimate and general relationships is among the most important aspirations we can reach for. It helps assure that our legacy will be that the world we leave behind will be a kinder, gentler, and more loving place.

Play It Forward

The most critical arena in which empathy needs to be practiced is in the care and raising of children. The health of future generations depends upon it. As older adults, our essential role in the raising of children is often overlooked, whether or not they are our own. The prevailing message is that once our own children are grown and having children of their own, our time in the sun has passed and our value in raising children has been drained away. The baton has been handed off to the next generation to raise the children while we, the older generation, no longer have a place or a purpose in child rearing of any sort. Neuroscience, however, tells us that nothing could be further from the truth.

Adults in the second half of life are critically important role models for children. Developmental theorists have identified the later stages of life as the time when creativity, moral thinking, problem solving, the softening of biases and prejudices, and various forms of self-acceptance all mature. Whether as parents of young adult children, grandparents, bosses, work colleagues, tutors, or athletic coaches, older adults play vital roles in shaping the worldviews of children as they prepare them not just to survive but actually to thrive in the world they will inherit.

Reverse mentoring is a recently coined term. It shifts the idea that skill acquisition is a one-way street that travels from elders to the young and inexperienced. Instead, reverse mentoring conveys the idea that skills acquisition in the workplace flows in both directions. Younger and older learn from one another and have different skill sets to offer each other. The reciprocal nature of that relationship increases the odds that empathy for each one's perspective will produce more diverse and successful solutions to the problems that are undertaken—in the workplace and in life.

Older adults also have the opportunity to model something not usually associated with them: playfulness. Playful adults are "active, adventurous, cheerful, energetic, friendly, funny, happy, humorous, impulsive, outgoing, sociable, spontaneous, and unpredictable," according to Yarnal and Quian.[29] To associate those attributes with older adults dispels the negative message that growing *old* equals growing *dull*. The attractiveness of these attributes invites the young to learn how to be a playful grown-up. Wanting to "know what it's like to be like" an older adult is a core ingredient in building empathy. Playfulness strengthens cross-generational connections. At the same time, maintaining playfulness throughout life counters the social disconnectedness and isolation that can ambush vital physical and emotional health in older adulthood.[30] Playfulness in older adults is one important quality that helps to shape children to become better able to let off steam. There is also a variety of health benefits enjoyed by people who are playful. An upcoming generation of children who are healthier, more resilient, and more creative in the face of life's stressors is a potent legacy![31]

Empathy in Action

Older adults have a wonderful opportunity to model one of the most important but overlooked aspects of empathy. *Prosocial* behavior (or *other-directed behavior*) is focused on ways of meeting or supporting the needs and wants of another person. In other words, prosocial behavior is empathy in action. The social benefits of empathic behavior have been known since the rise of civilization. More than two thousand years ago, Hillel, a first-century BCE scholar, was challenged by a cynic and skeptic to teach him the whole of Judaism's written laws while standing on one foot. Hillel responded to the challenge by stating, "Do not treat others in a way that you wouldn't want to be treated." Jesus later made a similar statement: "Do to others as you would have them do to you." Either way, the message is clear. We are not independent islands of individual people. We are interconnected beings, and the nature of our interactions shapes us and each other.

Empathy is our social glue. Empathy opens our hearts to others, connecting us to them and signaling that we are receptive and available to them. From the intimacy of connections to our long-term partners, to the deeply felt connections we form to the larger communities of which we are a part, empathy continues to play an important role in maintaining our physical and emotional health in the second half of life. What follows is a practice to help you build and strengthen your empathy circuits.

◇◇

A Helpful Practice

Painting an Open Heart:

A Meditation for Empathic Connection

You can read the following exercise, pausing as often as you choose. You can also find a recorded version of this exercise through our website (see Resources).

Sit in a comfortable position in a favorite chair. Allow your breathing to naturally slow down and deepen. Bring your awareness to the calming effect that tuning in to your breath has on your body and your mind. Stay with this cycle for several minutes. Breathing in and out. Slowly quieting the body as you calm the mind.

When ready, allow your eyes to close. Just keep breathing, gently quieting the body as you continue to calm your mind. By settling your mind and body, you have already begun to open your heart, making your brain more ready to rewire as you expand your empathy skills. Empathy allows you to feel inside of *you* what other people are feeling inside of *them*. Through empathy you can temporarily take on and take in another's experience so you can truly appreciate that person's perspective without judging it. Empathy creates a vital emotional link connecting another's feelings to your open heart.

Bring to mind the faces of the people you care deeply about. Select one person for whom you would like to develop more empathy. With whom would you like to develop a deeper and more satisfying relationship? With whom would you like to replace the baggage of negative feelings with a more positive and loving connection? Linger on the images and memories of time shared with that person. As you focus on that person's face and the times spent together, notice the emotions that rise up in your body. *How* do you become aware of them? What do you feel in your body? Notice the depth, the texture, and the tones of the feelings you connect with that person and your relationship.

Now imagine that you are an artist with a unique skill. You know how to mix and apply a special paint. Your paint creates empathy when you brush it on your heart. With your brush you open your heart to this other person. Your empathy brush allows you to feel that person's feelings as your own.

Apply the brush to your heart. Feel the other's love, sadness, hurt, or anger. With your open heart, you can meet that pain with forgiveness toward the other, with understanding of, patience with, and compassion for this person. In short, practice basic acceptance.

Each of us seeks to have our needs met, and we need one another to make that happen. We are not self-sufficient islands able to completely take care of ourselves all by ourselves. We need one another. Sometimes those needs are expressed in difficult ways. There may be times you've been hurt or offended by someone you care about. Even in recalling that, you may notice how those difficult feelings come back even now and how they affect your body. Notice those changes in your body. Don't judge them, but notice them.

Apply another layer of empathy paint to your heart. Feel your heart open even more. Let their feelings in, as difficult as that may be initially. Take their feelings in *as they feel them* while you remain receptive and open-hearted to them. As you do, the magic of empathy can expand. Your reaction to any negative feelings they've carried can soften. At the same time, by your remaining open without judgment to their feelings, the negativity they've been carrying can begin to soften too. Stay with the exercise, slowly reducing and transforming your tendency to react to any negative feelings by closing your heart. Replace your reactivity—the primary foe of empathy—with the ability to remain open-hearted to the other person even in the presence of negative emotions they may express. During the exercise, keep replacing any negative feelings that arise with another layer of paint from the empathy brush. Just hold that empathic space open. Keep breathing slow and steady. Anytime you find yourself wavering in your ability to maintain a heart open to the other person's feelings, apply another layer of the empathy paint and return your attention to your breathing.

With practice, your ability to hold empathy for the other can grow. It doesn't stop there, however. Regular practice of feeling empathy toward one person can help you become more empathic to many people.

The more empathic you become, the more confidently you can engage with the many people you encounter in your life. Regardless of their feelings, you can understand them and accept them as they are. You can use your empathy skills to build a stronger bridge between you and them that leads to a more cooperative and mutually beneficial relationship. Practicing empathy building can truly paint the years of the second half of life with a more golden hue.

11

A Youthful Brain Is Well Connected

Key 8

All real living is meeting.
—MARTIN BUBER

Key Points

- The need for social connection is hardwired into the human brain.
- The strength and type of social bond we form early in life has a lasting impact on our social bonds throughout life.
- Learning to create, grow, and maintain healthy social connections provides a protective health benefit, especially in the second half of life.
- Mental and physical health depend on how well our social connections provide us with meaning, purpose, and direction.
- The greatest measure of an individual's self-development is her or his social connections to others in the family, community, and wider society.

Our Primal Fear

Well into her late eighties, her husband long since gone, Bela was facing a move from the home in which she had raised her children and where she had lived alone for a number of years. She was going to an elder care facility in a new community, where she would be surrounded by people with similar backgrounds at a similar stage of life. She would have daily activities, aides, resources, and access to all manner of care. Yet as she considered the move, she made the poignant comment that she was "afraid to be alone there." Objectively, there was no basis for such a fear. She would hardly be alone for a minute during the day thanks to the carefully structured daily routine that would put her in touch with others.

The reality is that she wasn't talking about social isolation, which is the lack of actual physical contact with others. She was talking about loneliness, that psychological or existential sense of disconnection from others that is among the most primal and visceral fears we have. A psalm written more than twenty-five hundred years ago reflects this fear. The author, probably advanced in years, said, "Do not throw me away in my old age; do not abandon me when my strength fails."

Bela expressed that fear too. Her fear of loneliness reflected how powerfully our sense of connection can be formed to physical places and objects filled with potent memories (as her home was). Still, to face the existential fear of being alone and forgotten, we need dynamic, living, breathing relationships with others.

The Social Bond

There are powerful but hidden forces that influence our ability to form social bonds. For example, researchers led by Cristian Pasquaretta have shown that among social animals that are the "smartest" and most tolerant of one another (primates), you will also find brain networks within which information flows most efficiently. In other words, there is evidence from neuroscience that our social connections play a role in shaping our brains and enabling us to show more highly developed social behaviors.[1]

We are social animals. The smallest social group is the *dyad*, a group of two. The most basic dyad is a mother and child. A married or partnered pair of adults forms the elemental social unit around which larger social groups form. The strength of these bonds can last a lifetime, but they are tested by losses encountered in the second half of life. Thankfully, the bonds connecting us to others can be strengthened by developing the bonds that connect us more deeply to ourselves.

In one sense, the chemistry of our connection to others involves actual chemicals. Singer/songwriter Lou Reed's "Love Is Chemical" got it right. When chemical receptors in the brain's reward centers are flooded with tiny molecules called *vasopressin* and *oxytocin*, they generate strong urges to form lasting bonds.[2] Humans and other mammals that give attention to the care and raising of their offspring are the only creatures who have receptors sensitive to these bonding chemicals. Without them, there would be no long-term pair bonding. Without high levels of oxytocin, there would be no active nurturance of offspring by consistent parents.

Of course, social bonding involves more than molecules finding their receptor targets. Every one of the five senses is also involved in shaping the social bond. Most of us have heard of pheromones, the scent molecules that arouse amorous feelings toward potential mates. But pheromones don't act alone: all the senses get into the act of promoting social bonds.

Along the rocky shores of Antarctica, hundreds of thousands of Emperor penguins nest in communal rookeries. Each male-female pair lays one egg. While the females walk up to 120 miles to the ocean to feed and fatten up after laying their single egg, their male partners dutifully watch over their chicks in one of earth's harshest climates, patiently waiting their turn to walk to the sea upon their partner's return many weeks later. Loyal to a fault, these penguin pairs are able by their unique calls to recognize each other and their chicks from among the countless penguins walking about. For them, sound is the glue that cements their bonds.

The Imprint of Attachment

Our right brain is designed for pattern recognition, which occurs largely outside of our awareness. These patterns nevertheless strongly influence how we form relationships and with whom we form them.[3,4] The right brain notices what the conscious mind overlooks: voice patterns; habits of facial expression; arousal of emotions and which emotions tend to be dominant; expression of needs for love and intimacy. Ultimately, the right brain helps us learn what is safe and secure, guiding us so we can rapidly decide whether to approach or avoid a given encounter with others.

These are the fundamental elements of emotional attachment, and these patterns of attachment are set down quite early in life. Throughout the first years of life, the right brain is hard at work tracking and encoding these nonverbal, emotion-rich relationship patterns to learn what makes us feel safe and secure, what makes us feel wanted and loved, what encourages independence and confidence, and what signals threat and danger. Those early imprints stay with us over a lifetime, though they can be modified and shaped by our neuroplastic brain with mindful attention and persistent practice.

Social attachment patterns continue to play a central role in the second half of our lives. That doesn't change. What *does* change is our ability to bring awareness to the unwritten rules of those patterns and how they influence our daily choices. Through increased awareness of the relationship rules we carry, we become capable of composing new rules by which we can live more fully. We can pursue more satisfying and fulfilling connections to others that imbue the individuals' relationships with the capacity for richer emotional depth. And we can overcome any social limitations left over from early life experience.

Our relationships to others provide the social context within which we work out our relationship to ourselves. As David Wallin, a psychologist and expert in the field of attachment theory, says, relationships involve a "social biofeedback" system that enables us to learn to regulate our emotions.[5] In the process, we become better able to have our various emotional needs successfully met.

Wallin's research has focused on the importance of refashioning strong attachment bonds as a foundation for *psychological* health, but mounting evidence also shows the influences of social connection on *physical* health:[6]

- Our social connections shape the choices we make for how we maintain our health.[7]
- We tend to mimic the health behaviors (diet, weight control, exercise levels, smoking, and alcohol use patterns) of people in our social networks.[8]
- The shrinking of social networks results in health risks for aging.[9]
- Long-term caregiving of a chronically ill partner means a greater risk of illness for the caregiver.[10]

The Rewards of Social Connection

"The best thing we can do for our relationships with others, and with the transcendent, then, is to render our relationship to ourselves more conscious," writes James Hollis.[11]

Becoming more "conscious" about our reactions, our emotions, and our choices involves an everyday kind of enlightenment that has more to do with mental alertness and awareness than with world-changing insights. When you use the simple practices we have emphasized related to sleep, nutrition, exercise, flexibility, curiosity, and optimism, you will feel a positive shift in your relationship to yourself. Such practices open the door to improved relationships with others as well. Since we exist in "social biofeedback" networks, as Wallin noted, more open and intimate relationships to others reward us with greater abilities to improve our own health and well-being.

The more we build resilient connections to others, the better prepared we are to be emotionally grounded within ourselves. Then, when we face the inevitable disruption or loss of those relationships, we can rebound from those wounds more effectively. The ebb and flow between individuals connected through open minds and hearts enriches both of them, even in the face of loss. When we strengthen our personal and social connections, we become more able to accept whatever life brings us, while simultaneously tapping into life's joy. As C. J. Jung observed,

> I always thought that when we accepted things they overpowered us in some way or other. This turns out not to be true at all. . . . So now I intend to play the game of life, being receptive to whatever comes to me, good and bad, sun and shadow forever alternating, and, in this way, also accepting my own nature with its positive and negative sides. Thus everything becomes more alive to me.[12]

Accepting things as they are does not mean accepting that they will remain unchanged forever. The paradox is that in accepting things as they are in any given moment, we actually increase our capacity to make positive change in the *next* moment. We become capable of evolutionary growth, reflecting the slow and steady, step-by-step practice of one small change building on another.

Learning to accept the feedback we receive via our social network enables us to respond to the feedback with greater sensitivity, less defensiveness, and more compassion. Building healthy social connections this way can lead to a large-scale transformation of each person touched by those connections. Richer and more joyful relationships can emerge, further strengthening the social bonds.

There are many health consequences that can occur from having insufficient social bonds. For example, as recently as 2003, it was estimated that of the $1.3 *trillion* dollars that were spent in the United States on health care that year, at least 75 percent of that cost arose from health problems stemming from people's lifestyle choices.[13] Those unhealthy choices gave rise to obesity, diabetes, asthma, heart disease, and smoking and alcohol-related disease. The enormity of the problem has only grown since then.

We are not suggesting that all health care problems are caused primarily by a lack of social connectedness. After all, governmental and cultural choices involving air and water quality, farming regulations, health insurance coverage policies, and housing and educational subsidies have a huge impact too. Still, individual behavioral choices strongly influenced by the quality of your social connections to others contribute to these health problems as well. But why do people continue to engage in health-threatening behaviors when they know better? Why can't we change even when we want to?

We become more motivated to make behavioral changes when they are associated with deep personal meaning.[14] Research has found that people were more likely to make the changes that improved their health and increased their sense of well-being only when *internal* variables (such as self-esteem) were linked to the presence of *external* variables of social connection (such as a feeling of being loved). Meaning matters most when we are connected with others.

Ask yourself how you fare in each of the areas below, all of which support your moving from having the desire for change into actively working to change. Each area offers two statements. The first in each pair relates to social connection, while the second describes an associated internal quality.

1. I feel loved. / I have positive self-esteem.
2. I do not feel alone when I am making important decisions. / I have clear goals and plans.
3. I feel respected and listened to. / I am aware of my fears and anxieties.
4. I feel supported. / I have personal autonomy.
5. I am part of an environment where new learning opportunities are available. / I am challenged by questions to which I seek answers.
6. I trust the people in my life who care about me. / I trust myself.

The more you identify with the first statement in each statement pair, the more likely you are to be a part of a strong social network and experience the youthful brain rewards that go with it. If that isn't what you found, your answer can be a springboard to action to strengthen your connection to others.

The six paired statements in the list elevate our discussion by shifting the focus from an individual self to a self who is *embedded* in a network of social connections. The social self brings out the individual's highest potential to realize the greatest rewards. Most often, those rewards come from actions taken for the benefit of others.

Specifically, studies show that when facing what are called social dilemmas, offering a choice between doing something to benefit oneself or risking something to benefit another, most people say that they would choose the riskier but more altruistic (other-directed) option.[15] As we know, *saying* and *doing* are two different things. Therefore, this line of research was taken further. It explored, for example, what motivated people to donate a kidney to a stranger in need—a rather extreme form of altruism in action.

Initially, scientists were skeptical about what would motivate someone to undergo a serious operation to remove a healthy organ from their body and donate it to a total stranger. Psychologists were brought in to interview these potential donors to discover what must be wrong with them. The psychologists failed to find what they expected. They found something much more important instead. Their findings consistently showed that those individuals who actually donated a kidney were most likely to score highest on measures of self-esteem and reported feelings of overall well-being.[16] A new conclusion emerged: individuals blossom under the influence of positive social connectedness. Then, when that individual experiences an opportunity to act from their sense of meaningful connectedness, their actions often benefit others. The world's wisdom traditions have long advocated expressing our higher nature through service to others. Modern science provides solid evidence in support of this teaching.

Making Meaning Matter

The physician Victor Frankl was a towering figure. A practicing psychiatrist and researcher in Vienna prior to the outbreak of World War II, Dr. Frankl, his wife, father, mother, and brother were arrested and sent to Nazi concentration camps solely because they were Jews. Of that group, he was the only one to survive the war's horrors. In a world where human kindness seemed absent, as did the chances of survival, Dr. Frankl toiled daily to instill hope and counter deadly despair among the inmates of the death camps.

After liberation came in 1945, he translated his observations and discoveries into new therapies for which he became world-renowned. At the core of his work was recognition of the central role of meaning and purpose in life. He proposed that not only do meaning and purpose enrich life, but the absence of meaning and purpose can actually shorten life. He recognized that life is about more than surviving. In his book *The Unheard Cry for Meaning*, he wrote, "The truth is that as the struggle for survival has subsided, the question has emerged: survival for what? Ever more people today have the means to live, but no meaning to live for."[17]

Among the greatest responsibilities of the second half of life is to answer Frankl's call and challenge: What is the meaning and purpose for which you live? This question is being asked by an increasing number of aging baby boomers. The old paradigm assumed that when you reach a certain age, it is time to step off the stage of life. Like the waves lapping at the shore, each generation has its moment to make a splash before it recedes, its energy spent, to make room for the next wave coming up from behind.

The new paradigm is different. This paradigm suggests eighty is the new sixty. Increasing life expectancies support this. As Frankl observed, the means to live cannot substitute for the reasons to live. Aging boomers are heeding the call and, as author Marc Freedman outlined in his book *Encore*, they are discovering their personal second acts in life. Freedman's research found that people entering their fifties share several things in common that are relevant to social connection as a path to spurring positive social action.[18]

- They view their lives as having an active career phase beyond traditional retirement age.
- They seek second careers at higher rates than ever before.
- What they seek is less driven by money and more focused on finding meaning and purpose.
- Becoming less interested in *making more*, they seek opportunities to *make a difference*.

Wayne Muller, a therapist and minister, focused on the call for meaning in a different way.[19] Unlike Freedman's focus on finding meaning through action, Muller looked at the emergence of mental and emotional clarity about who we are on the inside, a clarity that lets us better manifest that inner self in the outer world. He focused on four questions, which we invite you to ask yourself. Set aside some quiet, uninterrupted time to contemplate or meditate on them. Allow yourself to develop satisfying answers by revisiting the questions over time. The four questions are

- Who am I?
- What do I love?
- How shall I live, knowing I will die?
- What is my gift to the family of the earth?

Return to the four questions repeatedly. Each time, the response you discover can mature and become more heartfelt. The questions are not meant to be a pop quiz that you answer once, hand in, and move on to the next chapter. They are a blueprint for a solid foundation on which to build a life of meaning. The building requires ongoing and attentive refinement. As you can readily see, Muller's questions, like Freedman's, lead from inner self to outer world, from the individual to the larger social world of which each of us is an integral and essential part.

Most faith traditions have emphasized how precious our all-too-short lives can be. Most faith traditions have also emphasized that as individuals we are most alive when we are acting in service of others and the world we share with them. There seems to be a universal principle that is found in all the faith traditions and thereby transcends them. This philosophical perspective goes beyond the individual to see the individual as part of a larger (perhaps divine?) whole.

The Hindu greeting *namaste* means, "I bow to the divine in you." To view one another through this lens immediately subdues our tendency to evaluate and judge one another when we meet. *How do you look (compared to me)? Are you happy (compared to me)? Are you struggling with something upsetting (more than me)? Are you as successful, established, recognized, well-liked, etc. (compared to me)?* By subordinating that tendency to judge, evaluate, and compare, and at the same time acknowledging that each of us is much more than the physical sum of our parts, we transform the way we meet one another. We become able to greet each other as equals who enrich one another through the encounter.

Building a Meaningfully Connected Life

A key stepping stone to youthful aging is to refine who we are and how we function as socially connected beings. How do we do that? How do we transform our encounters with one another into meetings between two inspired beings eager to do with each other and do for others what we might be unable to do on our own? The next section outlines steps you can take. First, some necessary background.

In the late 1800s a young man was born in Vienna, Austria. His mother, without explanation or forewarning, abandoned him and the family when young Martin Buber was just three years old. His overworked and traumatized father sent young Martin to be raised by his grandparents. The connection to those loving grandparents may well have saved Martin's life. His early attachment experiences—the positive *and* the negative—may also have served to fashion his lifelong interest in understanding the nature of relationships. The culmination of his life of study was published in his world-famous book *I and Thou.*[20]

For those unfamiliar with this work, here is a brief summary. Buber described two primary types of relationships: I-Thou and I-it. The ideal is the I-Thou relationship in which both parties are fully present to each other. Through the sharing of that fully attentive presence, both parties are elevated. Both parties acknowledge the *namaste* or divine spark in the other. Both parties come away feeling heard, validated, and affirmed. I-Thou translates the singular *I* into a plural interpersonal experience: "*We* exist, *we* matter, and *our* sharing of *our* lives makes sense!"

Buber wrote, "All real living is meeting." He was referring to the deep level of connection that comes when people meet each other at the I-Thou level. We have all had the experience, no matter how fleeting, of interacting with someone who seemed to be attentively listening to us with an open heart, and how it generated stirrings within us to respond in kind. This is the kind of encounter that can happen as easily between intimate partners in fifty-year-long relationships as between strangers who interact with each other for those few short moments on a bus, a plane ride, or at the checkout line at the grocery store. What is required is the active effort of showing up as you are, with mind and heart open to influence, and being influenced by the encounter with the other. As we've seen, empathy allows us to read the other and to be read by the other. In an I-Thou encounter, empathy flows. When coupled with the mutual reading of each other's inner states, the social bond is strengthened. The various health benefits of the social bond are activated. The door to individual and mutual joy, fulfillment, and satisfaction is opened.

I-it encounters, on the other hand, involve either no mutual presence or the experience of being alone in the physical presence of another. The I-it encounter isn't about interacting with another person so much as standing back apart from them while acting toward them, seeking what they have to offer you. In an I-it encounter:

- The clerk *should* complete the transaction quickly so you can be quickly on your way to your important next appointment.

- The teller *should* complete the withdrawal quickly because what you have to do is important, you are important, and time is money.
- The friend on the phone is wasting your time by attempting to share something with you. Feelings of impatience arise in you as you wait for them to pause. They *should* recognize *your* needs. Then, you can start saying what you have been waiting to say, disregarding what they are saying so you can use them as your dumping ground for what you want to get off your chest.

The I-it encounter makes the other the object to you as the subject. When the shoe is on the other foot, we know how it feels. We sense when we have been the object. When treated as a physical object, we often describe the experience in physical language. "I felt small." "I felt kicked aside." "I felt like a piece of garbage." As objects, we are no longer in a true two-way interaction, since I-it encounters are largely one-way streets. We have value only so long as the other is getting what they want from us. Then, like that piece of garbage, we are tossed aside and left saying, "I felt completely used!" These are all comments that reflect the failure of that encounter to rise to Buber's level of an I-Thou meeting.

As mental health clinicians with more than fifty years of clinical practice between us, we have borne witness countless times to the transformative power of the I-Thou relationship to shape people's lives. Many times, with tears in their eyes, our clients have said to us, "This is the first time I have really felt listened to." That experience of real living as real meeting (paraphrasing Buber's words) was a telling moment for these clients. Having their lives witnessed by a caring other was a key moment in the blossoming of their human potential. Social connectedness, particularly in life's second half, helps us to get there in the face of the challenges of illness, retirement, losses of loved ones and friends, and most especially the awareness of our own mortality, which becomes more keenly felt.

Social Connectedness in Action

Older adults with strong and active social networks have a 50 percent increase in survival.[21] Isn't that a strong motivator to learn how to build, sustain, or improve existing connections to others? For the 20 percent of older adults actively involved in caring for an ill spouse, it often becomes hard to remain connected to larger social networks. Isolation and loneliness rates skyrocket when people in long-term caring relationships become disconnected from their larger social lives.[22] Brother William Geenen has said about these twin afflictions that "isolation and loneliness are the malnutrition of the aging."[23] A wide range of experts in many aging-related fields recognize this and agree that the challenges involved are not just about living longer but also living *better*. They have identified a number of important steps that support individuals' efforts to stay connected.

Research undertaken by Emlet and Moceri[24] addresses the physical challenges of aging by focusing on what it takes to build age-friendly communities. They found several key elements that support greater social connectedness:

- We need to build communities that attend to the kinds of physical challenges identified by the AGNES research (as we saw in chapter 10, AGNES involved wearing suits to mimic for young people the experience of getting about in an older body).
- We need to build in social roles that emphasize *mutual benefit* (creating I-Thou communities). In age-friendly

communities, older adults are not seen simply as recipients of services and consumers of resources generated by the young. Older adults in age-friendly communities are highly valued as people who make important contributions to the community through active involvement in a range of activities that can include volunteerism, tutoring/teaching, and mentorship. They are valued as important positive role models of what younger people can grow up to become.

- The youthful older adult was found to be a lifelong learner. Satisfying the curiosity of older adult minds was associated with the maintenance of agile brains well into advanced age for all but those suffering from dementia. Whether the learning setting is a book group, a Bible-study group, an informal community education class, or a formal course offered through a recognized educational institution, the opportunity to engage in group-based learning is an important path to deeper connections to others.

- At the other end of the continuum is the importance of playtime. Study after study continues to rediscover the importance of play as we age.[25] The cultivation of a number of ways to use leisure time, especially when leisure activities link us to others, clearly confers health benefits that go beyond raising your bowling score or lowering your eighteen-hole golf handicap. Take your playtime seriously! Enjoy it fully.

- Healthy aging and social connectedness also depend upon our developing effective plans to self-manage illness as much as possible. Self-management does not mean doing things entirely on your own. Instead, illness self-management involves doing what you can for yourself when feasible but also clearly understanding when and how to access various supportive resources to address your health needs. The self-management of health involves three steps: *First, be proactive about your health.* You will need the motivation to take appropriate steps to manage your health along with the self-esteem necessary to perceive that those efforts are worthwhile. *Second, develop health literacy.* Learn how an illness impacts you so you can minimize factors that worsen the condition while taking steps to maximize your return to optimal health. *Third, create strong relationships with your health care team.* The very idea of a "team" already implies social connection. You and your provider call the shots together. Together you set any action in motion and decide when additional resources are needed. As a team, you can take the time to decide together about what actions should be taken to impact your health. Actions taken together can account for your whole-person needs and not just focus narrowly on a particular body part. We recognize that finding someone who is able and willing to fulfill that partnership role is not always easy. The rewards of doing so should not be underestimated.

The Circle of Life

Each of us began our lives connected to someone else. The umbilical cord was literally the lifeline that sustained us until we were ready to enter the world. From the moment the cord was cut, we were launched in two directions simultaneously. None of us has ever stopped seeking ways to bring those two directions together again. None of us will ever fully succeed in those efforts.

On the one hand, the cutting of the cord heralds the precise moment when we begin our journey to individual autonomy and self-sufficiency. While we may rely on others at times, the drive for independence is strong and is intimately connected to how we grow a sense of *self*-esteem, *self*-confidence, and *self*-direction. On the other hand, the cord cutting heralds the beginning of our never-ending search to connect to another in ways that provide the security and comfort that we once "knew" while we were ripening in the womb. We spend our lives searching for the ideal partner, a person who can perceive our needs and wants almost intuitively, without our having to ask. The ways in which the simultaneous searches for separateness and union are pursued are as numerous as the people undertaking this essential journey. There is no one right path. There is no ideal balance. Nevertheless, this chapter has highlighted core elements that you can combine to reach that balance in ways unique to you.

We have described how the urge to connect with others helps us to buffer primal fears of being cut off and alone in the world. That fear is often at its strongest in the second half of life, sometimes intensifying with each passing year. At the same time, developing our ability to connect with and listen to our most deeply felt personal passions helps to enliven the connections we ultimately form with others. The discovery of meaning and purpose is intimately tied to how well we can construct I-Thou encounters with others.

George Bernard Shaw conveyed the spirit of connection through service. Heeding his words takes you one step closer to the creation of a purpose-driven life:

> This is the true joy in life, the being used for a purpose recognized by yourself as a mighty one; the being a force of nature instead of a feverish selfish clod of ailments and grievances complaining that the world will not devote itself to making you happy.
>
> I am of the opinion that my life belongs to the whole community and as long as I live it is my privilege to do for it whatever I can. I

want to be thoroughly used up when I die, for the harder I work, the more I live. I rejoice in life for its own sake. Life is no "brief candle" to me. It is sort of a splendid torch which I have a hold of for the moment, and I want to make it burn as brightly as possible before handing it over to future generations.

◇◇

A Helpful Practice
An Exercise in Meaning Making

Your great mistake is to act the drama
as if you were alone.
Put down the weight of your aloneness and ease into
the conversation.
Everything is waiting for you.
  —David Whyte[26]

Earlier in this chapter we presented the four questions developed by Wayne Muller. We close with a second set of four questions. The two sets may ultimately help you to reach the same place, to tap into your heart to access the elements from which your future life can be built.

When you sit down to contemplate these questions, the above words of poet David Whyte can help you to focus. Use your focused attention skills to tune in to your deeper wisdom and tune out extraneous distractions. Then, as the insights and answers gradually come into focus, take action. Take the steps to help transform your potential into your lived practice.

1. What do I most deeply want to experience?
2. What do I most deeply want to express?
3. What do I most deeply want to create?
4. What do I most deeply want to contribute?

Using the focused attention skills you have been developing throughout the book, ask yourself one question at a time, and then focus on the thoughts and feelings that arise for 2–5 minutes. Jot down the thoughts and go on to the next question, taking each one in turn until you have finished with all four questions. Repeat this several times a week over the next several weeks.

12

A Youthful Brain Is Authentic

Key 9

Be who you are. That is all that you ever volunteered for.
Be who you are, that is all that was ever required.
Be who you are, that is all that was ever needed.
Be who you are.

—BARBARA BRENNAN

Key Concepts

- Becoming a fully embodied, loving, and authentic self is life's great work, for which we are all still in training.
- The seeds of true self may be found in any of life's experiences, including what we deem successes *and* failures, triumphs *and* tribulations.
- A vital brain, a vibrant mind, and an open heart allow for the possibility of awakening to true self, but they do not guarantee it. We must still learn to listen deeply, discern wisely, and honor courageously the yearnings of the still, small voice within.

Reb Zusya, a righteous rabbi, lay dying. His disciples surrounded him and were astounded to see that their teacher and sage, a man whom all regarded as a model of appropriate thought and deed, shook with fear at the prospect of death and judgment.

"Master," said his disciples, "why do you fear God's judgment? You have lived life with the faith of Abraham. You have been as nurturing as Rachel. You have feared the Divine as Moses himself. Why do you fear judgment?"

Zusya took a deep, shuddering breath, and replied, "When I come before the throne of judgment, I am not afraid that God will ask, 'Why were you not more like Abraham?' After all, I can say, 'O God, you know best of all that I am Zusya, not Abraham. How then should I have been more like Abraham?' And if God should ask, 'Why were you not more caring, like Rachel?' I can respond, 'Master of the Universe, you made me to be Zusya, not Rachel. If you wanted me to be more like Rachel, you should have made me more like Rachel.' And should the True Judge say, 'Zusya, why were you not more like Moses?' I can respond, 'O Mysterious One, who am I, Zusya, that I should be like Moses?' But I tremble in terror, because I think the Eternal will ask me another question. I believe I will be asked, 'Zusya, why were you not more like Zusya?' And when I am asked this, how shall I respond?"

The above is a Hasidic tale, graciously shared in this version by Rabbi David Kominsky, who summarized the story's lesson in this way: "We seek not to become the perfect person, but to be the person we are meant to be."[1]

To become the person we are meant to be may seem a simple thing. "How could I be anyone else?" you may ask. For others, it might feel daunting. "What does that mean, exactly, to be the person we are meant to be? And just how am I supposed to find out what that is?"

For most of us, becoming fully one's self is not an easy task. There is no direct pathway laid out for us by science or self-help or even, necessarily, religion. Becoming the person you were meant to be involves deep inner work, and there are no clear guidelines for it since it is a journey we must each make on our own. And yet, is there any more important pursuit than to be fully, deeply, authentically one's self? When all is said and done, is there really any other game in town?

We view this journey toward a fully embodied, authentic self as the work of a lifetime. There is no end to it while we are alive, because we are always changing, and each new moment and circumstance calls upon us in fresh ways. Everything we have written in this book so far prepares us for this task, creating the conditions for such fulfillment, *but not guaranteeing it.*

We humans have freedom of choice, after all. Strange though it may seem, we can choose *not* to be fully ourselves, and most of us do so most of the time. We seek to please others. We compare ourselves to others. We diminish ourselves. We value other pursuits more highly. We refuse to awaken and see things as they are. The result, as the Zusya story points out, is that *we can fail to live our own lives.*

In this final chapter, we wish to offer you guidance, of a sort, for how to claim the fullness of your own life, no matter your age, your current state of health, or what you may perceive as past failures. The good news is that, so long as we are living and breathing, there is still time to awaken to true self. There is still time.

Know Who You Are: Awakening to True Self

Now I become myself. It's taken
Time, many years and places;
I have been dissolved and shaken,
Worn other people's faces . . .
—May Sarton

"What a long time it can take to become the person one has always been," writes Parker Palmer in *Let Your Life Speak.* "How often in the process we mask ourselves in faces that are not our own. How much dissolving and shaking of ego we must endure before we discover our deep identity—the true self within every human being that is the seed of authentic vocation."[2]

Who among us has not worn other people's faces, living out the expectations of a parent, a teacher, or a friend, trying so hard to be someone we're not? Who among us has not felt their identity shaken, unsure who they really are or how to move forward and retain a sense of self? Think about your life for a moment. When did *you* begin to forsake yourself, and what prompted you to do so?

Speaking with a group of seventh graders recently, we saw clearly that for them, this process was already well under way. We were discussing depression, something they knew a lot about, and sadly much of that knowledge seemed to come from personal experience. But even more surprising was the source of their struggle. One after another, these children said the same thing in different words: that they suffered from the weight of expectations. By age thirteen, they were learning the pain of "wearing other people's faces."

Parker Palmer points out that this connection to true self is a frequent casualty of childhood, and one of the core tasks of aging is to reclaim the birthright gifts of true self: "We are disabused of original giftedness in the first half of our lives. Then—if we are awake, aware, and able to admit our loss—we spend the second half trying to recover and reclaim the gift we once possessed."[3]

Consider this story by Portia Nelson that illustrates how we might wake up in stages to our own lives:

Autobiography in Five Short Chapters
Chapter 1
I walk down the street.
There is a deep hole in the sidewalk.

I fall in.

I am lost . . . I am helpless.

It isn't my fault.

It takes forever to find a way out.

Chapter 2

I walk down the same street.

There is a deep hole in the sidewalk.

I pretend I don't see it.

I fall in again.

I can't believe I am in the same place.

But it isn't my fault.

It still takes a long time to get out.

Chapter 3

I walk down the same street.

There is a deep hole in the sidewalk.

I see it is there.

I still fall in . . . it's a habit.

My eyes are open.

I know where I am.

It is my fault.

I get out immediately.

Chapter 4

I walk down the same street.

There is a deep hole in the sidewalk.

I walk around it.

Chapter 5

I walk down another street.[4]

If this story makes us laugh, it is because we recognize ourselves in it, and our own folly. We have all fallen into the same holes, made the same mistakes, repeated the same foolish things that didn't work the last ten or twenty or hundred times we tried them. A good psychotherapist or spiritual director can help shorten the time it takes to wake up and see what we are doing, but whether we enlist a guide or go it alone, we do at some point have to awaken to our own lives, to see clearly where we are and to accept the pain and loss that have been part of our journey. Indeed, it might be through the pain and loss that we awaken. Where do you see yourself in the story? What chapter are you in at this time in your life?

There are three essential skills required of us to discover true self, skills that we have been working toward throughout this book:

- We must be able to clearly see what is (cultivate the quality of *awareness*).
- We must be able to face that truth without flinching (embrace the quality of *honesty*).
- And we must be able to read what is written in our own heart (sharpen the quality of *discernment*).

These qualities are not a given, nor are they easy to achieve. But each of us possesses the innate skills needed to achieve them. Indeed, we have been honing them our entire lives through our precious life experiences, any of which can be the means of our own awakening. Three of the most effective pathways for awakening to true self come directly from life experience: *suffering* (which is inevitable); *joy* (which is a choice); and *longing* (which is often hidden).

The Road Most Traveled: Awakening through Pain

Most of us are like the person in the story above: it's not until we've fallen into the same hole multiple times, each time causing some kind of suffering, that it begins to dawn on us that we don't have to keep doing this. There are as many varieties of struggle as there are people: we each have our own experience in this regard. But no matter the form it takes, our pain, loss, or unhappiness can be a cause for awakening. It may be wise to embrace it rather than to resist it.

The abstract nature of these ideas calls for a real-life example. I (Dr. Emmons) will use my own story simply because it is the story I know best and is, therefore, for me most authentic. This is a story of vocation, which many can relate to since work and livelihood take up so much of our time and energy. But the process of awakening can happen in any area of life, whether you are working or not, young or old.

One of the first signs that I was not living my own life was that I entered college and declared myself a predentistry student. I had no interest whatsoever in dentistry, but I greatly admired a dentist from my hometown and thought I wanted to be like him. I quickly realized that choice was a mistake and changed course, but only a little. I became premed because it seemed an easy transition (I was good at science) and because everyone I knew thought it was such a great profession, one I would be good at: "We need people like you in medicine," they said. I did not stop to ask whether *I* thought it was right for me or whether it was something I *wanted* to do. Lacking sufficient awareness, I stepped into a stream that carried me along with greater and greater force, and one that I met with greater and greater resistance.

The signs that I was not following my own path could hardly have been more obvious. Even then I was aware of my heart sinking when I received my acceptance letter to medical school; of my classmates seeming to be so much more grateful than I to be there; of the loss of a love for learning and my tepid effort in my classes. Three times I tried to quit and go to seminary or grad school in one of the humanities. But my parents and everyone else I knew seemed so pleased with what I was doing (and disapproving of my floundering efforts to get out) that I willingly suppressed my own growing feelings of discontent. And I continued to do so for the next fifteen years!

The pain of shutting down my own voice made an already difficult training that much harder. Living day to day with so much internal resistance proved a high cost to pay for wearing other people's faces. That is *not* a path I would recommend to anyone. But it was my path.

Within a few scant years of starting my psychiatric practice, working in a medical model in which I was skilled but still conflicted, I had developed all the signs of professional burnout (a term that seems to diminish the depth and richness of the experience). My instincts, my personal experience, my heart (in other words, my *authentic self*) all told me to do something different, to practice more holistically, to focus more on health and resilience than on disease. But the nature of the business of health care, and my own complicity in it, made it very hard for me to see a different path. I knew that I was unhappy, that's for sure, but I didn't know how to change that fact. I felt as if I were in Dante's *Inferno*, lost in the middle of this road I called my life.

Still, the unhappiness was enough to wake me up. One day I finally conceded that I couldn't keep going on as I was. I decided to quit my job and take a new path, no matter what it required from me. I would like to say that it was courage that allowed me to take that leap, to leave behind a secure job and a sure income for something completely unknown. But it was not really courage—it was just that I came to the point that I could no longer *not* do it. In other words, I had grown so tired of living a divided life, of leaving so much of my self out of my work, that I had no real choice but to bring the more authentic parts of myself into my role as a psychiatrist. At least I had no choice if I didn't want to continue to feel so unhappy. And I didn't.

We all have our stories, and we need to honor them. We need to bring our inner lives out of shadow, into the light of personal and communal reflection. We need to live divided no more, and an honest grappling with our struggles can get us there. But the path of suffering is not the only way to get there, and it is certainly not the easiest or the most enjoyable way. There is also the path of joy.

Follow Your Bliss: Awakening to Joy

Joseph Campbell, the great mythologist, became known for his famous phrase: "Follow your bliss." By this, he did not mean that we are to become self-centered or self-absorbed. He was telling us to wake up to the joy that is all around, and to let that joy, or bliss, be a guide for how to live our lives. "Awe is what moves us forward," he said. Mary Oliver expressed a similar sentiment in her poem "When Death Comes": "When it's over, I want to say: all my life / I was a bride married to amazement."[5]

Seeing that joy is all around us, living a life filled with awe, being married to amazement—it sounds so grand, and no doubt it would be, if only we could do it. The great poets continually bring us back to such possibilities, and we continually deny them. Perhaps the very grandness of this vision leaves us feeling that it is beyond our reach.

Yet it is not beyond our reach; it is just our thinking that makes it appear so. For example, we tend to look at our life in its entirety and think that it should be grand in a very particular way—usually some vision we adopted from other people, from popular culture or religion—but not in the way that it is. We could, however, choose to honor the life that we're actually living, and to see it in much smaller fragments, as a series of little bits that might add up to something grand over time.

We are given continual opportunities to choose, and it is the accumulation of these small choices that determines what our lives become. Each of us must decide, in every moment, how to use our time, where to place our energy, how to think or act, what to see or to ignore. Even if we seem to live in a world of sorrows, joy is all around us, if we could only see it, if we would make the choice to live in joy. That is easier said than done; yet it can be done. It is not a onetime decision that lasts forever. It is best done in increments, one moment at a time.

When I left my job, I was unable to be guided by joy, because I could not yet see or feel it. I decided to take a year's sabbatical and retool myself. I then studied what I'd always been drawn toward, the things that I naturally loved but hadn't seemed to me to be very doctor-like: diet, fitness, natural therapies, and mindfulness and spiritual practices.

These had always been the stuff of my life, much closer to my true nature than the masks I wore with such resistance through my training and first few years of psychiatric practice. Since that moment of decision, now nearly twenty years ago, I have gradually embraced the things that come so naturally to me, while not turning completely away from the role of physician (which I now find fits me when it is integrated with these other approaches). Surprisingly, the greatest change has been not in the content of what I do, but rather in the growing feeling that I bring more and more of my *self* into my work. I am becoming myself.

It is not as if I have experienced a continuous series of bliss-filled moments since then. I have those moments, to be sure, but overall there is a feeling of normalcy, a sense that I am just being myself in a way that feels natural and good to me. But it is nothing special, and that sometimes confuses people as to whether they are on the right track. We have been conditioned to think that being our truest (our "highest") self is something exceptional, out of the ordinary, and that we will feel some intensely positive emotion when we achieve it. My experience is that it can be quite ordinary and it doesn't necessarily involve any special or intense emotions. Yet it is among the most satisfying states in which one can live.

It is deeply gratifying (blissful) when you find that being yourself is *enough*, and when you know that offering that to the world makes it somehow a better place. Indeed, giving back seems to be a central ingredient for joy—offering yourself to the world freely, without reserve. You may or may not be compensated for it (financially, at least), but it needs to be done nonetheless, and what comes back to you is more joy. It is not something to keep to yourself. It is something to be shared with the world, as Joseph Campbell knew so well:

> *You must return with the bliss and integrate it.*
> *The return is seeing the radiance is everywhere.*
> *Sanctify the place you are in.*
> *Follow your bliss.*

The Still, Small Voice: Awakening through Longing

There is a third pathway to awakening to true self, perhaps less common than the others not because it is rare, but because it involves a depth of listening that few of us sufficiently honor. That is the path of *longing* or yearning. This moves us into the territory of spirituality and the concept of *soul*, known by some as "the still, small voice." Not everyone believes in the existence of the soul, or perhaps they define it differently than we do, but we think it is real and welcome the sense of mystery that still surrounds it.

The soul often speaks through a quiet inner voice, hard to hear or understand if we are not listening carefully, and easy to misinterpret if we are not skilled at discernment. But understanding it needn't be overly complicated either. All that is required is to turn our attention toward it and listen deeply.

My own attempts to heed this voice were born out of a sense that there was something missing or askew in my life. Not knowing what it was or what to do about it, I still honored my belief that perhaps the answer lay within. I had no training or any models in my life for how to attend to this, so I sought out help. Not far from where I did my medical training

there was a Benedictine monastery, and though I wasn't Catholic, I began to go there for retreats. There, I learned to be still, to do contemplative practices, and to listen within. Later, I entered spiritual direction, and later still, I trained in mindfulness and other forms of meditation. Slowly, I learned how to listen to the inner voice. But I haven't always done so.

For several years, I chose to ignore what that voice was telling me. Either I didn't believe it, or I didn't want to hear what it had to say. So it got louder and more insistent. It began to speak through my body, which started to break down despite my being young and fit. I developed recurrent sinus infections, and then asthma-like symptoms including tight, constricted breathing.

Finally, I decided to pay attention. I sat down on my meditation bench and invited my highest self to speak, consciously agreeing to listen and abide by what it had to say. I then asked the question, "Should I leave this job?" and I noticed my airways open up. I couldn't believe it, so I asked the question in a different way: "Should I stay in this job?" My airways closed. Still not trusting it, I went through this sequence three more times, and each time it was the same: yes, airways opened; no, airways closed. The clarity of the message, along with my conscious commitment to heed my own deeper self, allowed me to break through my fear and take the action I knew I needed to take.

This inner voice never goes away. If we can't sense it, perhaps it's because we have turned our attention away from it; or we have chosen to suppress it (as I did for fifteen years); or the din of our day-to-day busyness simply makes it impossible to hear. Yet the voice of longing is ever-present and ready to come forth when invited, *so long as it is safe to do so*. It speaks the language of the heart, the language of story, music, poetry. It unfailingly draws us toward goodness, toward that which is of our higher nature. It *always* has our best interest at heart (which is undoubtedly in the best interest of others as well). Its nuances are as varied as the human beings who receive them, but the essence of its

message seems to boil down to one great desire that is shared by all: the longing for connection, to love and be loved.

Listening to this inner voice is often a deeply personal experience, best undertaken in quiet, private moments. But it can also come forth in relationship to others when the conditions are right: when there is a sense of safety, an open invitation, and no attempt to fix or judge. Below we offer two means for listening to this voice; one turns our attention inward, and the other outward. Both add value, and combining them may offer the most effective means of discernment.

<><><><><><><><><><><><><><><><><><><><><><><><><><><><><><><><><><><><><><>

A Helpful Practice

Turning toward the Self: The Inner Practice of Deep Listening

- Find a quiet space and time for personal reflection, when you are sure to be alone, awake, and alert.

- Sit quietly and allow your mind to be still. It may help you to focus on your breath for a few moments, or to notice the fact that you are sitting and how you are grounded by it.

- Silently hold the intention that you wish to listen and be guided by your inner voice, the part of you that is with you always and continuously draws you toward your highest good.

- Hold a question in your mind if you have one. If you have no burning questions, you can simply hold the desire to see what is arising for you at this moment in your life.

- Make no effort to answer the questions or figure anything out. Let go of the notion that something profound or important has to happen. Simply create the space to be with your deeper self, much as you would with a dear friend.

- See yourself as a curious observer, wondering what might arise, but with no attachment to it. Look for a felt experience, a quick-

ening of the heart, a sense of opening, warmth, or movement. Words may arise, or pictures, memories, or sensations. Keep sitting, with your awareness placed lightly wherever it seems to be drawn in your body. Usually, that is near the heart or the gut, or somewhere in the midsection of the body.

- If you have a specific choice to make or dilemma to resolve, you can phrase it in the form of a yes/no question and observe the response. When you hold the answer yes, what happens in your body? When you hold a no, what happens? Make no judgments about this; just keep observing with interest and a sense of not knowing.

- If you'd prefer, you can hold an open-ended question, such as "How can I focus my energies on what is most important for me now?" or "How will I know whether this is the right path for me?" Or better yet, phrase your own question. Then just hold the question lightly and observe whatever you experience without judgment.

- Whenever it feels right to you, you may wish to write some of your observations in a journal. Try to stay focused on describing your experience, rather than drawing conclusions from it or analyzing the experience. You may do that later.

- Return to this inner listening often. As with any relationship, the more time and attention you give it, the richer and more meaningful it becomes.

Turning toward Others: The Shared Practice of Deep Listening

- Gather two or more trusted people with the express purpose of genuinely listening to one another. They may include friends or family members, but take care that their ideas of who you are or what you should do aren't held too strongly. You want to choose people who can allow your true self to come forth, without judgment or preconceived ideas.

- This may be done at a time when you need discernment, when the way forward is unclear to you; or it may be done at any time simply to allow your inner voice to be spoken aloud, to be brought into the light of day.

- Set aside an hour or more and seek to ensure that there will be no interruptions.

- Allow one person to be the center of focus (it's okay to start with yourself). If there is sufficient time, each participant may have the opportunity to speak. If not, set up another time for others to be the focus person, so that you don't rush the experience. Spaciousness of time is a requirement for the inner voice to come out.

- When you are the speaker, do your best to speak from the heart, without the need to entertain or to impress or to present yourself in any certain light. Seek to present the unfiltered version of what you believe to be true, without interpretation, analysis, or the need to say what you think the others wish to hear.

- When you are the listener, just listen. Set your own story aside. Refrain from the desire to interpret what is said or to offer counsel or support, or even to share something similar from your own life. Try to limit yourself to asking *only* authentic questions (about something you really wonder about), rather than asking a question that you think you know the answer to or attempting to lead the focus person to a certain conclusion.

- Let there be periods of silence. Remember that the still, small voice speaks only under the most safe and inviting conditions. Wait for it, allowing rather than cajoling. You don't need to fill the moments of silence. They are ripe with opportunity.

- Likewise, if painful emotions arise, just allow them to be, with no need to stop them or even to offer comfort. The emotions may need to be felt.

- Maintain a stance of acceptance and compassion. We are all in this together. We all have our blind spots and vulnerabilities, right alongside our deep wisdom and strength.

- Honor the preciousness of what is shared. It needn't be deep or profound or conclusive. Speaking the inner voice aloud into the world allows the speaker to hear it much more clearly. As a listener, honor the speaker's confidentiality. Do not talk about what was shared, even with the person who shared it, unless that person asks you about it later.

◇◇◇

Live Who You Are: Following True Self

There's a thread you follow. It goes among
things that change. But it doesn't change.
—William Stafford

As the story goes, a woman named Nadine Stair, age eighty-five, was asked what she would do differently if she had her life to live over again. Her response included, "I'd dare to make more mistakes next time . . . I would take more chances . . . I would perhaps have more actual troubles, but I'd have fewer imaginary ones." She listed several choices she would make to be more daring, like eating more ice cream and climbing more mountains, and concluded with the wish to reach for more beauty: "I'd pick more daisies."[6]

It does take courage, after all, to live an authentic life. You may be signing up for more actual troubles (though it would also be nice to have fewer imaginary ones). Stepping fully into your own life involves risk and vulnerability. So why do it?

Signs of an Authentic Life

How do you know when you are living from true self? What do you get from it? Below are seven signs of an authentic life, which also reveal some of its paybacks:

1. **Flowing.** You may still put in a great deal of effort toward your goals, but there is a sense of ease about it, a naturalness that makes it seem less like work and more like play.

2. **Self-Acceptance.** Knowing the truth of who you really are, that you are not broken but whole, frees you from the need to strive or achieve or meet expectations. You can then hold yourself with kindness.

3. **Vulnerability.** You can allow yourself to be open and vulnerable, to take more chances, because you feel more secure in yourself and in the outcome.

4. **Savoring.** When you stop rejecting some aspects of your experience, you can draw more pleasure from those that you enjoy. You can pick more daisies.

5. **Appreciation.** Gratitude arises naturally, without trying, when we live from our true center. As a side benefit, it also makes us healthier and happier.

6. **Meaning.** Meaning flows naturally from self-expression, from bringing your unique voice, abilities, and creativity into the world. These are meant to be manifest, to be shared with others, rather than kept to oneself.

7. **Equanimity.** When you stop resisting what is, when you no longer grasp some things and push others away, you are left with a feeling of deep calm. You know the deep truth that all will be well.

Follow the Thread

A line from a Leonard Cohen song puts into poetic language the experience of losing one's connection with true self: "The blizzard of the world has crossed the threshold and it has overturned the order of the soul."

Living in the wintry part of this country, it's not hard to imagine "the blizzard of the world." We all experience storms, inner and outer, large and small, which unsettle our lives and take us off course, "overturning the order of the soul." Life is never a straight path. It veers and darts, and we will at times lose our way along with the connection to authentic self. It is inevitable. The only questions are, How long will it take to get back onto our own path, and how do we do so?

If you grew up on a farm in a wintry climate, you might remember seeing a rope tied on one end to the barn, and on the opposite end to the back door of the house. If the farmer had to go to the barn in the midst of a blizzard, the tethered rope would guide him safely back home. This image offers a potent metaphor for the inner life. There is a rope, a thread that follows us throughout our lives, offering guidance back to true self when we get lost or are caught in a storm. How do you know it exists? Usually a reflection on your own life journey will reveal it.

Look back over your life, especially at the nodal points, those moments you can see in the rearview mirror that were filled with risk, potential, or change. No doubt you will see themes emerge, certain constants of preference, means, or purpose. We all have our own ways of approaching the challenges and opportunities that life offers, and our own reasons behind what we do. It just takes a little inner exploration to tease them out.

◇◇

Consider these questions to help gain insight into the thread *you* follow:

- When are you most on path, feeling most at home? What are you doing; who are you with; what do you feel; what are you like?
- What are the constants in your life? For instance, what values guide your decisions? What sustains you in times of challenge

or loss? What shows up during major transitions and choice points?

- What is it that draws you out of the storms? Describe the hearth that beckons you or the home that you would like to return to.

<hr>

It is useful to reflect on such things, but don't feel as if you have to figure this out once and for all. It is not really necessary to answer these questions definitively. The thread is there whether you can see it or not, and the answers may keep changing anyway. All that is really needed is to keep paying attention, to remain mindfully aware, and to keep asking your self, moment by moment, "What is the next right thing?"

This is rather like using a satellite GPS guidance system to get you where you want to go. It's nice to see the overview, but all you really need to know is your very next turn. And when you stop paying attention and make a wrong turn, your internal GPS can take your new location, recalibrate, and get you back on track.

Wayne Muller states this idea beautifully in his book *A Life of Being, Having, and Doing Enough*: "When we listen for, and surrender to, the simple clarity of the next right thing—liberated from the inevitability of previous plans or declarations—we are likely to find that the next moment brings with it a sense of easy sufficiency. By feeling our way along this path, moving carefully into the absolutely perfectly next right thing, we are more likely to do less, move more slowly, and come upon some completely unexpected meadow of spacious, gentle time and care that feels remarkably, for now, like enough."[7]

We can let out a collective sigh: "Ah, that is enough. This moment is enough. I am enough." Be who you are. That is all that is needed from you.

Resources for Staying Sharp

Dr. Emmons and Dr. Alter are available for speaking engagements, retreats, and workshops. They can be reached through www.stayingsharp.org.

Practices for Developing the 9 Keys for a Youthful Brain

Staying Sharp Program

Developed by Drs. Emmons and Alter, this is a hands-on, step-by-step training to bring to life the concepts in this book. For more information or to sign up for the program, go to www.stayingsharp.org.

CDs, DVDs

We offer a series of CDs and DVDs with guided meditations, nutritional programs, and exercises for staying sharp. Go to www.stayingsharp.org for a complete listing.

Nutritional Supplements for Healthy Aging

Customized, pharmaceutical-grade nutritional supports for healthy mood, sleep, and vital aging are available online through the Lifestyle Pharmacy at www.staying sharp.org.

Mindfulness-based Stress Reduction Training

This training, typically offered in eight weekly sessions, is one of the best methods for developing attention skills. Check in your area for MBSR teachers or mindfulness meditation instructors.

Lumosity

This is a computer-based set of exercises that are presented as games but which have been shown to improve attention and working memory skills.

Healing Rhythms

This is a fifteen-step, home-based biofeedback program that teaches an important set of self-care and self-regulation skills, including improving selective attention.

CogMed Training

This is a training approach offered by health professionals, usually psychologists/neuropsychologists. It is a structure program that trains attention and working memory skills.

Hypnosis/Guided Imagery Training

Many health professionals are able to teach you self-hypnosis and guided imagery that you can use on your own. Being able to direct your mind using these approaches helps you rewire your brain for greater optimism. Look for clinicians trained by credible organizations such as the American Society of Clinical Hypnosis (ASCH), the Society for Clinical and Experimental Hypnosis (SCEH), the International Society for Hypnosis (ISH), or the Milton Erickson Foundation.

Medication

For certain individuals, prescription medication can be useful to improve attention and prime you for greater success in daily life.

Nutritional Supplementation

Individuals sensitive to prescription medication or who simply prefer not to pursue that route can find measurable benefit through the use of specific nutritional/herbal supplements that work on the attention systems of the brain (refer to chapter 6).

Books

Arden, J. 2010. *Rewire Your Brain: Think Your Way to a Better Life*. New York: John Wiley & Sons, Inc.

Arrien, A. 2007. *The Second Half of Life: Opening the Eight Gates of Wisdom*. Louisville, CO: Sounds True.

Chödrön, P. 2012. *Living Beautifully with Uncertainty and Change*. Boston: Shambhala Publications.

Cope, S. 2012. *The Great Work of Your Life: A Guide for the Journey to Your True Calling*. New York: Bantam Books.

Dement, W. 2000. *The Promise of Sleep: A Pioneer in Sleep Medicine Explores the Vital Connection between Health, Happiness, and a Good Night's Sleep*. New York: Dell.

Doidge, N. 2007. *The Brain That Changes Itself: Stories of Personal Triumph from the Frontiers of Brain Science*. New York: Penguin Books.

Duhigg, C. 2012. *The Power of Habit*. New York: Random House Publishers.

Emmons, H. 2006. *The Chemistry of Joy*. New York: Simon & Schuster.

Emmons, H. 2010. *The Chemistry of Calm*. New York: Touchstone Books.

Hollis, J. 2005. *Finding Meaning in the Second Half of Life: How to Finally, Really Grow Up*. New York: Gotham Books.

Johnson, R. and J. Ruhl. 2007. *Living Your Unlived Life: Coping with Unrealized Dreams and Fulfilling Your Purpose in the Second Half of Life*. New York: Tarcher Penguin Publishers.

McTaggart, L. 2011. *The Bond: Connecting Through the Space Between Us*. New York: Free Press.

Merzenich, M. 2013. *Soft-Wired: How the New Science of Brain Plasticity Can Change Your Life*. San Francisco: Parnassus Publishing.

Moody, H. 1998. *The Five Stages of the Soul: Charting the Spiritual Passages that Shape Our Lives*. New York: Anchor Books.

Muller, W. 1996. *How, Then, Shall We Live? Four Simple Questions That Reveal the Beauty and Meaning of Our Lives*. New York: Bantam Books.

Naiman, R. 2006. *Healing Night: The Science and Spirit of Sleeping, Dreaming, and Awakening*. Minneapolis: Syren Book Publishing.

Nepo, M. 2005. *The Exquisite Risk: Daring to Live an Authentic Life*. New York: Three Rivers Press.

Nepo, M. 2012. *Seven Thousand Ways to Listen: Staying Close to What Is Sacred*. New York: Atria Paperback.

Palmer, P. 1999. *Let Your Life Speak*. New York: Jossey-Bass Publishers.

Palmer, P. 2004. *A Hidden Wholeness: The Journey toward an Undivided Life*. New York: Jossey-Bass Publishers.

Schachter-Shalomi, Z. 1997. *From Age-ing to Sage-ing: A Revolutionary Approach to Growing Older*. New York: Time Warner Books.

Sharot, T. 2012. *The Optimism Bias: A Tour of the Irrationally Positive Brain*. New York: Vintage Books.

Smalley, S. and D. Winston. 2010. *Fully Present: the Science, Art, and Practice of Mindfulness*. Boston: Da Capo Press.

Todd, R. 2008. *The Thing Itself: On the Search for Authenticity.* New York: Riverhead Books.

Trungpa, C. 2009. *Smile at Fear: Awakening the True Heart of Bravery.* Boston: Shambhala Publishers.

Walsh, R. 1999. *Essential Spirituality: The 7 Central Practices to Awaken Heart and Mind.* New York: John Wiley & Sons, Inc.

Weil, A. 2007. *Healthy Aging: A Lifelong Guide to Your Well-being.* New York: Anchor Books.

Products

Relaxing Rhythms Biofeedback Training Program. Available at www.wilddivine.com /relaxing-rhythms-software-iol.html.

The HeartMath Institute. Offers multiple levels of biofeedback-based training products for stress management, emotional regulation, and sleep restoration. www .hearthmath.com.

Acknowledgments

Henry Emmons, MD:

This book feels like a natural outcome of my lifetime to date, and it raises gratitude for all the mentors, teachers, and supporters who have given of themselves so richly and generously. I am especially mindful of the many shining examples of how to age well, with grace and dignity, no matter what challenges or losses are encountered along the way. If you look for them, you will find these sages all around you.

I am continually grateful to Janis Vallely, my literary agent, whose wise guidance and support have made it possible for me to be an author, and who has touched so many lives with the books she has helped manifest over her highly successful career. And I feel so fortunate to work again with Michelle Howry, senior editor at Simon and Schuster, who has shepherded this book into publication. I am so appreciative of the attentiveness, skill, and grace that she brings to her work.

Thanks once again to my friends and colleagues with Partners in Resilience, Sandra Kacher and Carolyn Denton, for their ongoing support and reading of the manuscript; and Susan Bourgerie for her skillful and courageous early editing. This book is unquestionably better for her hand in it.

David Alter, you have been a steady friend and a brilliant colleague for more than a quarter of a century now. It has been a joy to work on this book together and to capture a small part of the curiosity, enthusiasm, and passion that you so clearly offer the world. Here's to another quarter century of creative collaboration!

And finally, thank you to the many good people who have entrusted their care to me over the years. I echo the sentiment of Pema Chödrön: "How did I get so lucky to have my heart awakened to others and their suffering?"

David Alter, PhD:

The physical writing of this book has been the final step of a much longer process, the beginning of which I can scarcely glimpse. In many ways, the book is merely a tangible expression of what life has been teaching me all along, but which I had yet to fully appreciate. The writing has been like assembling a 10,000-piece jigsaw puzzle of seemingly disconnected life experiences that ultimately come together to reveal a coherent picture. For me, there have been several key puzzle pieces that I want to specifically acknowledge.

From conception to completion, this project has been carefully stewarded by Janis Vallely and Michelle Howry. Their thoughtful and respectful hands helped assure that this project remained on task, on target, and expressing the appropriate voice. Having a gifted editor as a sister-in-law was a bonus that paid continuous dividends. Thank you, Mindy Werner.

Being raised in a family that valued learning and discovery sharpened my sense of curiosity, and for that I am indebted to my grandparents and parents. Having siblings taught me the importance of connection and play, and for that I remain forever grateful to my wonderful sister and brothers. For 35 years, I have basked in the trust and unflinching support of loving in-laws who have immersed me in an extended family, which has so formed my character. I have been blessed to have friendships that have spanned decades, and those friends have occupied many positions: They have been confidants in life's darkest moments. They have been cheerleaders and coaches, urging persistence when the incline was steep. They have shown wicked sarcasm and brutal honesty when I've stepped out of line in ways that threatened to have me forget my place in my world. And they have laughed deeply with me as we've encountered so many ways in which life is truly comical in its capacity for constant surprise. I especially want to express my appreciation to Gil Mann. Through countless get-togethers, he freely gave his time and wise counsel that not all that glitters is gold, and that through patient and persistent focus, something polished and enduring can emerge.

The following three people are unaware of the depth of the impact they have had on me. Still, I want to acknowledge Ben Blom, PhD, my professor who, more than any other, opened my eyes to the potential for positive change that lies within us, awaiting the alchemy that transforms potential into lived expression. I want to thank Jeff Zeig, PhD, a teacher, an author, a mentor, and a friend, who helped me appreciate that words have the power to evoke novel experiences that help people change their lives for the better. Finally, I want to thank Rod Fraser, a friend who taught me through living his example, that the messages we convey to you in this book keep life fresh, fulfilling, and forever forward-looking.

Henry Emmons, MD is my coauthor and dear friend. Sometimes two voices joined together are not simply louder. They are also clearer and more resonant in a way that creates harmonious sound. I want to thank you for your gentle and steady influence, which so consistently helped to fashion and refashion this work.

Special acknowledgment has to go to Zach, Jonathan, and Rachel, my three children. They inspire me and instill in me a deep-felt sense that the future is in good hands. Each is following a different path in their lives. And yet, each invests their unique path with courage, open-heartedness, and generosity of spirit that will, I trust, serve them well in the years to come. To Jodi: my partner, my muse, my love, and my hope, whose trust and support of my vision has never wavered, I am forever indebted. And lastly, to the bizarre and tragic condition we call "dementia," which has stolen my father's memory from him, and with it much of the essence of the man who taught me so much. While the book may have been written anyway, my close encounter with dementia instilled in the writing an intimacy and urgency that I believe made the writing better.

Notes

2. The Brain That Time Built

1. P. Whitehouse, *The Myth of Alzheimer's: What You Aren't Being Told about Today's Most Dreaded Diagnosis* (New York: St. Martin's Press, 2008).
2. P. Greenwood and R. Parasuraman, *Nurturing the Older Brain and Mind* (Cambridge, MA: MIT Press, 2012).
3. R. D. Fields, *The Other Brain: From Dementia to Schizophrenia, How New Discoveries about the Brain Are Revolutionizing Medicine and Science* (New York: Simon & Schuster, 2009).
4. I. McGilchrist, *The Master and His Emissary: The Divided Brain and the Making of the Western World* (New Haven: Yale University Press, 2009).
5. http://www.immersionactive.com/resources/50-plus-facts-and-fiction.
6. Pew Research Center for the People and the Press, poll, Dec. 15, 2010.
7. Y. Taki et al., "Voxel-Based Morphometry of Age-Related Structural Change of Gray Matter for Each Decade in Normal Male Subjects," paper presented at the Ninth Annual Meeting of the Organization for Human Brain Mapping, New York City, 2003.
8. E. Goldberg, *The Wisdom Paradox* (New York: Gotham Books, 2006).
9. P. Greenwood and R. Parasuraman, "Ameliorating Cognitive Aging: A Neurocognitive Framework," chap. 4 in *Nurturing the Older Brain and Mind* (Cambridge, MA: MIT Press, 2012).
10. Greenwood and Parasuraman, p. 5; Goldberg, p. 11.
11. D. Snowdon et al., "Linguistic Ability in Early Life and Cognitive Function and Alzheimer's Disease in Later Life," *JAMA* 275, no. 7 (1996): 528–33.

3. The Power of Attention

1. D. J. Simons and C. F. Chabris, "Gorillas in Our Midst: Sustained Inattentional Blindness for Dynamic Events," *Perception* 28, no. 9 (May 1999): 1059–74.
2. E. R. Graham and D. M. Burke, "Aging Increases Inattentional Blindness to the Gorilla in Our Midst," *Psychology and Aging* 26, no. 1 (Mar. 2011), 162–66.
3. G. Mark et al., "The Cost of Interrupted Work: More Speed and Stress," *Proceedings of the SIGCHI Conference on Human Factors in Computing Systems* (2008): 107–10.

4. C. Woolston, "Multitasking and Stress," *HealthDay* (Mar. 2013): http://con sumer.healthday.com/encyclopedia/article.asp?AID=646052.

5. Quoted by C. Rosen, "The Myth of Multitasking," *The New Atlantis* 20 (Spring 2008): 105–10.

6. E. Ophir et al., "Cognitive Control in Media Multitaskers," *Proceedings of the National Academy of Sciences of the United States of America* 106, no. 37 (Sept. 15, 2009): 15583–87.

7. P. Grossman et al., "Mindfulness-Based Stress Reduction and Health Benefits: A Meta-Analysis," *Journal of Psychosomatic Research* 57, no. 1 (2004): 35–43.

8. N. E. Morone et al., "Mindfulness Meditation for the Treatment of Chronic Low Back Pain in Older Adults: A Randomized Controlled Pilot Study," *Pain* 134 (2008): 310–19.

9. H. Cramer et al., "Mindfulness-Based Stress Reduction for Breast Cancer: A Systematic Review and Meta-Analysis," *Current Oncology* 19, no. 5 (2012): 343–52.

10. R. J. Davidson et al., "Alterations in Brain and Immune Function Produced by Mindfulness Meditation," *Psychosomatic Medicine* 65 (2003): 564–70.

11. J.D. Creswell et al., "Mindfulness Meditation Training Effects on CD4+ T Lymphocytes in HIV-1 Infected Adults: A Small Randomized Controlled Trial," *Brain, Behavior, and Immunity* 23, no. 2 (Feb. 2009): 184–88.

12. M. Killingsworth, "Does Mind-Wandering Make You Unhappy?," *Greater Good*, July 16, 2013, http://greatergood.berkeley.edu/article/item/does_mind_wander ing_make_you_unhappy.

13. W. Hasenkamp et al., "Mind Wandering and Attention during Focused Medita- tion: A Fine-Grained Temporal Analysis of Fluctuating Cognitive States," *Neuro- Image* 59 (2012): 750–60.

14. W. Hasenkamp, "How to Focus a Wandering Mind," *Daily Good*, July 17, 2013. http://greatergood.berkeley.edu/article/item/how_to_focus_a_wandering_mind.

15. F. Zeidan et al., "Mindfulness Meditation Improves Cognition: Evidence of Brief Mental Training," *Consciousness and Cognition*, 19, no. 2 (June 2010): 597-605.

16. L. Bylsma et al., "A Meta-analysis of Emotional Reactivity in Major Depressive Disorder," *Clinical Psychology Review*, 28, no. 4 (Apr. 2008): 676–91.

17. J. Lutz et al., "Mindfulness and Emotion Regulation—an fMRI Study," *Social Cognitive and Affective Neuroscience*, doi:10.1093/scan/nst043 (first published online Apr. 5, 2013).

18. E. Luders et al., "The Underlying Anatomical Correlates of Long-Term Medita- tion: Larger Hippocampal and Frontal Volumes of Gray Matter," *NeuroImage*, 45 (2009): 672–78.

19. E. Luders, quoted by M. Wheeler in "How to Build a Bigger Brain," *UCLA News*, May 12, 2009, http://newsroom.ucla.edu/portal/ucla/PRN-how-to-build -a-bigger-brain-91273.aspx.

20. J. Johnson, H. Emmons, et al., "Resilience Training for Depressed and Stressed Healthcare Professionals," Jan. 2014 (submitted for publication).

4. A Youthful Brain Loves Movement: Key 1

1. B. Winter et al., "High-Impact Running Improves Learning," *Neurobiology of Learning and Memory* 87, no. 4 (2007): 597–609.

2. J. S. Snyder et al., "The Effects of Exercise and Stress on the Survival and Matu-

ration of Adult-Generated Granule Cells," *Hippocampus*, Epub ahead of print (Jan. 20, 2009): 1–9, doi:10.1002/hipo.20552.

3. S. Vaynman and F. Gomez-Pinilla, "License to Run: Exercise Impacts Functional Plasticity in the Intact and Injured Central Nervous System by Using Neurotrophins," *Neurorehabilitation and Neural Repair* 19, no. 4 (2005): 283–95.

4. http://www.cdc.gov/physicalactivity/everyone/guidelines/adults.html.

5. Center for Disease Control and Prevention, "One in Five Adults Meets Overall Physical Activity Guidelines," Press Release, May 2, 2013, http://www.cdc.gov/media/releases/2013/p0502-physical-activity.html.

6. N. Mischel et al., "Physical (In)activity-Dependent Structural Plasticity in Bulbospinal Catecholaminergic Neurons of Rat Rostral Ventrolateral Medulla," *Journal of Comparative Neurology* 522, no. 3 (Feb. 15, 2014): 499–513.

7. A. Gow et al., "Neuroprotective Lifestyles and the Aging Brain: Activity, Atrophy, and White Matter Integrity," *Neurology* 79, no. 17 (Oct. 2012): 1802–8.

8. K. I. Erickson et al., "Exercise Training Increases Size of Hippocampus and Improves Memory," *Proceedings of the National Academy of Sciences* 108, no. 7 (Feb. 15, 2011): 3017–22.

9. J. Mota-Pereira, J. Silverio, et al., "Moderate Exercise Improves Depression Parameters in Treatment-Resistant Patients with Major Depressive Disorder," *Journal of Psychiatric Research* 45, no. 8 (Aug. 2011).

10. J. B. Bartholomew et al., "Effects of Acute Exercise on Mood and Well-Being in Patients with Major Depressive Disorder," *Medicine and Science in Sports and Exercise* 37, no. 12 (2005): 2032–37.

11. Alzheimer's Association, "2013 Alzheimer's Disease Facts and Figures," www.alz.org/downloads/facts_figures_2013.pdf, accessed Jan. 25, 2014.

12. G. Small et al., "Healthy Behavior and Memory Self-Reports in Young, Middle-Aged, and Older Adults," *International Psychogeriatrics* 25, no. 6 (June 2013): 981–89.

13. R. Carrington et al., "Cardiorespiratory Fitness and Accelerated Cognitive Decline with Aging," *Journals of Gerontology*, doi:10.1093/gerona/glt144 (first published online Nov. 5, 2013).

14. D. Head et al., "Exercise Engagement as a Moderator of the Effects of APOE Genotype on Amyloid Deposition," *Archives of Neurology* 69, no. 5 (2012): 636–43.

15. K. Liang et al., "Exercise and Alzheimer's Disease Biomarkers in Cognitively Normal Older Adults," *Annals of Neurology* 68, no. 3 (2010): 311–18.

16. E. J. Huang and L. F. Reichart, "Neurotrophins: Roles in Neuronal Development and Function," *Annual Review of Neuroscience* 24 (Mar. 2001): 677–736.

17. X. Jiang et al., "BDNF Variation and Mood Disorders: A Novel Functional Promoter Polymorphism and Val66Met Are Associated with Anxiety But Have Opposing Effects," *Neuropsychopharmacology* 30 (2005): 1353–61.

18. H. S. Phillips et al., "BDNF mRNA Is Decreased in the Hippocampus of Individuals with Alzheimer's Disease," *Neuron* 7, no. 5 (Nov. 1991): 695–702.

19. D. W. Howells et al., "Reduced BDNF mRNA Expression in the Parkinson's Disease Substantia Nigra," *Experimental Neurology* 166, no. 1 (Nov. 2000): 127–35.

20. J. L. Warner-Schmidt and R. S. Duman, "Hippocampal Neurogenesis: Opposing Effects of Stress and Antidepressant Treatment," *Hippocampus* 16, no. 3 (2006): 239–49.

21. H. van Praag et al., "Running Increases Cell Proliferation and Neurogenesis in the Adult Mouse Dentate Gyrus," *Nature Neuroscience* 2 (1999): 266–70.
22. A. A. Garza et al., "Exercise, Antidepressant Treatment, and BDNF mRNA Expression in the Aging Brain," *Pharmacology, Biochemistry and Behavior* 77, no. 2 (2004): 209–20.
23. B. Eadie et al., "Voluntary Exercise Increases Neurogenic Activity in the Dentate Gyrus of the Adult Mammalian Brain: Fact of Fiction?" poster presented at the Annual Meeting of the Society for Neuroscience, 2004.
24. L. Byberg et al., "Total Mortality after Changes in Leisure-Time Physical Activity in 50-Year-Old Men: 35-Year Follow-Up of Population-Based Cohort," *British Medical Journal* 338 (2009): b668, doi:10.1136/bmj.b688.
25. I. Barnett et al., "Changes in Household, Transport and Recreational Physical Activity and Television Viewing Time across the Transition to Retirement: Longitudinal Evidence from the EPIC-Norfolk Cohort," *Journal of Epidemiology and Community Health,"* doi:10.1136/jech-2013-203225.
26. B. Liebman, "Chair Today, Gone Tomorrow," interview with James Levine, MD, *Nutrition Action Healthletter* 35, no. 3 (Apr. 2008): 3–6.
27. B. Ainsworth, W. Haskell, et al., "2011 Compendium of Physical Activities: A Second Update of Codes and MET Values," *Medicine and Science in Sports and Exercise* 43, no. 8: 1575–81 (2011).
28. Heydari et al., "The Effect of High-Intensity Intermittent Exercise on Body Composition of Overweight Young Males," *Journal of Obesity* 2012, article ID 480467 (2012), http://dx.doi.org/10.1155/2012/480467.
29. J. King, "A Comparison of the Effects of Interval Training vs. Continuous Training on Weight Loss and Body Composition in Obese Pre-Menopausal Women," M.A. thesis, East Tennessee State University.
30. P. Wahl, "Hormonal and Metabolic Responses to High Intensity Interval Training," *Journal of Sports Medicine and Doping Studies* 3, no. 1 (2013): e132, doi:10.4172/2161-0673.1000e132.
31. J. Gillen et al., "Acute High-Intensity Interval Exercise Reduces the Postprandial Glucose Response and Prevalence of Hyperglycaemia in Patients with Type 2 Diabetes," *Diabetes Obesity and Metabolism* 14, vol. 6 (June 2012): 575–77.
32. Heydari et al., "The Effect of High-Intensity Intermittent Exercise on Body Composition of Overweight Young Males," *Journal of Obesity* (2012), article ID 480467, 8 pp. http://dx.doi.org/10.1155/2012/480467.

5. A Youthful Brain Is Well Rested: Key 2

1. http://www.cdc.gov/features/dssleep.
2. National Institutes of Health, "National Institutes of Health State-of-the-Science Conference Statement on Manifestations and Management of Chronic Insomnia in Adults," *Sleep* 28 (June 2005): 1049–57.
3. M. Wang, S. Wang, and P. Tsai, "Cognitive Behavioral Therapy for Primary Insomnia: A Systematic Review," *Journal of Advances in Nursing* 50 (2005): 553–64.
4. www.sleepfoundation.org/article/sleep-related-problems/sleep-aids-and-insomnia.
5. www.sleepfoundation.org/article/sleep-topics/aging-and-sleep.
6. B. Carey, "Sleep Therapy Seen as an Aid for Depression," *The New York Times*, Nov. 18, 2013, accessed Feb. 20, 2014.
7. C. Carney et al., "The Relation between Insomnia Symptoms, Mood, and Rumi-

nation about Insomnia Symptoms," *Journal of Clinical Sleep Medicine* 9, no. 6 (June 15, 2013): 567–75.

8. J. Suttie, "Why You Should Sleep Your Way to the Top," *Greater Good*, Dec. 1, 2013, accessed Feb. 20, 2014. http://greatergood.berkeley.edu/article/item/why_sleep_your_way_top.

9. S. Brand et al., "Adolescents with Greater Mental Toughness Show Higher Sleep Efficiency, More Deep Sleep and Fewer Awakenings after Sleep Onset," *Journal of Adolescent Health* 54, no. 1 (Jan. 2014): 109–13.

10. J. Suttie, "Why You Should Sleep Your Way to the Top," http://greatergood.berk eley.edu/article/item/why_sleep_your_way_top.

11. B. Mander et al., "Prefrontal Atrophy, Disrupted NREM Slow Waves and Impaired Hippocampal-Dependent Memory in Aging," *Nature Neuroscience* 16, (2013): 357–64.

12. J. Suttie, "Why You Should Sleep Your Way to the Top."

13. A. Prather et al., "Gender Differences in the Prospective Associations of Self-Reported Sleep Quality with Biomarkers of Systemic Inflammation and Coagulation: Findings from the Heart and Soul Study," *Journal of Psychiatric Research* 47, no. 9 (Sept. 2013): 1228–35, doi:10.1016/j.jpsychires.2013.05.004. Epub 2013 Jun 5.

14. J. Broussard et al., "Impaired Insulin Signaling in Human Adipocytes after Experimental Sleep Restriction," *Annals of Internal Medicine* 157 (2012): 549–57.

15. Y. Liu et al., "Association between Perceived Insufficient Sleep, Frequent Mental Distress, Obesity and Chronic Diseases among US Adults, 2009 Behavioral Risk Factor Surveillance System," *BMC Public Health* 13 (2013): 84, no. l, doi:10.1186/1471-2458-13-84.

16. A. Jagannath et al., "Sleep and Circadian Rhythm Disruption in Neuropsychiatric Illness," *Current Opinion in Neurobiology* 23, no. 5 (Oct. 2013): 888–94.

17. F. Benedetti and M. Terman, "Much Ado About . . . A Moody Clock," *Biological Psychiatry* 74, no. 4 (Aug. 15, 2013): 236–37.

18. C. Moller-Levet et al., "Effects of Insufficient Sleep on Circadian Rhythmicity and Expression Amplitude of the Human Blood Transcriptome," *Proceedings of the National Academy of Sciences* 110, no. 12 (Mar. 19, 2013): 1132–41.

19. K. Obayashi et al., "Exposure to Light at Night and Risk of Depression in the Elderly," *Journal of Affective Disorders*, article in press.

20. R. Lieverse et al., "Bright Light Treatment in Elderly Patients with Nonseasonal Major Depressive Disorder: A Randomized Placebo-Controlled Trial," *Archives of General Psychiatry* 68, no. 1 (2011): 61–70, doi:10.1001/archgenpsychiatry.2010 .183.

21. A. Wirzjustice et al., "Chronotherapeutics (Light and Wake Therapy) in Affective Disorders," *Psychological Medicine* 35 (2005): 939944, doi:10.1017/S003329170500437X.

22. J. Gooley et al., "Exposure to Room Light before Bedtime Suppresses Melatonin Onset and Shortens Melatonin Duration in Humans," *Journal of Clinical Endocrinology and Metabolism* 96, no. 3 (Mar. 2011): E463-472.

23. L. Xie et al., "Sleep Drives Metabolite Clearance from the Adult Brain," *Science* 342, no. 6156 (Oct. 18, 2013): 373–77.

24. B. Luscombe, "Your Brain Cells Shrink While You Sleep (And That's a Good Thing)," *Time*, Oct. 17, 2013, accessed Feb. 23, 2014, http://healthland.time

.com/2013/10/17/your-brain-cells-shrink-while-you-sleep-and-thats-a-good -thing/#ixzz2uBRM9BAD.

6. A Youthful Brain Is Well Nourished: Key 3

1. Q. Yang et al., "Added Sugar Intake and Cardiovascular Diseases Mortality among US Adults," *JAMA Internal Medicine* 2014, doi:10.1001/jamain ternmed.2013.13563.

2. R. Chowdhury et al., "Association of Dietary, Circulating, and Supplement Fatty Acids with Coronary Risk: A Systematic Review and Meta-analysis," *Archives of Internal Medicine* 160, no. 6 (Mar. 2014): 398–406.

3. http://well.blogs.nytimes.com/2014/03/17/study-questions-fat-and-heart -disease-link/?_php=true&_type=blogs&_r=0.

4. www.gallup.com/poll/165671/obesity-rate-climbing-2013.aspx.

5. K. Duffy and B. Popkin, "Energy Density, Portion Size, and Eating Occasions: Contributions to Increased Energy Intake in the United States, 1977–2006," *PLoS Medicine*, 2011, doi:10.1371/journal.pmed.1001050.

6. G. Vistoli et al., "Advanced Glycoxidation and Lipoxidation End Products (AGEs and ALEs): An Overview of Their Mechanisms of Formation," *Free Radical Research* 47, no. 12 (Aug. 2013): Supplement 1: 3–27.

7. S. Shaikh et al., "Advanced Glycation End Products Induce in Vitro Cross-Linking of Alpha-Synuclein and Accelerate the Process of Intracellular Inclusion Body Formation," *Journal of Neuroscience Research* 86, no. 9 (July 2008): 2071–82.

8. C. Carvalho et al., "Increased Susceptibility to Amyloid-β Toxicity in Rat Brain Microvascular Endothelial Cells under Hyperglycemic Conditions," *Journal of Alzheimer's Disease* 38, no. 1 (Oct. 2013): 75–83.

9. N. Cherbuin et al., "Higher Normal Fasting Plasma Glucose Is Associated with Hippocampal Atrophy: The PATH Study," *Neurology* 79, no. 10 (Sept. 4, 2012): 1019–26.

10. P. Crane et al., "Glucose Levels and Risk of Dementia," *New England Journal of Medicine* 369 (Aug. 8, 2013): 540–48.

11. R. Wilson et al., "Proneness to Psychological Distress Is Associated with Risk of Alzheimer's Disease," *Neurology* 61 (2003):1479–85.

12. L. Tsai and R. Madabhushi, "Alzheimer's disease: A Protective Factor for the Ageing Brain," *Nature* 507 (Mar. 27, 2014): 439–40, doi:10.1038/nature13214.

13. M. Parrott and C. Greenwood, "Dietary Influences on Cognitive Function with Aging: From High-Fat Diets to Healthful Eating," *Annals of the New York Academy of Sciences* 1114 (2007): 389–97.

14. A. Rubio-Tapia et al., "Increased Prevalence and Mortality in Undiagnosed Celiac Disease," *Gastroenterology* 137, no. 1 (July 2009): 88–93, doi:10.1053 /j.gastro.2009.03.059.

15. A. Vajdani, "The Characterization of the Repertoire of Wheat Antigens and Peptides Involved in the Humoral Immune Responses in Patients with Gluten Sensitivity and Crohn's Disease," *ISRN Allergy* (Oct. 27, 2011), doi:10.5402/2011 /950104.

16. S. Collins et al., "The Adoptive Transfer of Behavioral Phenotype via the Intestinal Microbiota: Experimental Evidence and Clinical Implications," *Current Opinion in Microbiology* 16, no. 3 (June 2013): 240–45.

17. G. Clarke et al., "The Microbiome-Gut-Brain Axis during Early Life Regulates the Hippocampal Serotonergic System in a Sex-Dependent Manner," *Molecular Psychiatry* 18, no. 6 (June 12, 2012): 666–73, doi:10.1038/mp.2012.77.

18. T. Dinan et al., "Psychobiotics: A Novel Class of Psychotropic," *Biological Psychiatry* 74, no. 10 (Nov. 15, 2013): 720–26.

19. J. Bravo et al., "Ingestion of *Lactobacillus* Strain Regulates Emotional Behavior and Central GABA Receptor Expression in a Mouse via The Vagus Nerve," *Proceedings of the National Academy of Sciences* 108, no. 38 (2011): 16050–55, doi:10.1073/pnas.1102999108.

20. J. Markle et al., "Sex Differences in the Gut Microbiome Drive Hormone-Dependent Regulation of Autoimmunity," *Science* 339, no. 6123 (Jan. 17, 2013): 1084–88, doi:10.1126/science.1233521.

21. Helmholtz Centre For Environmental Research—UFZ, "GI Tract Bacteria May Protect against Autoimmune Disease," *ScienceDaily*, Jan. 17, 2013.

22. M. Houston, "The Role of Nutrition and Nutraceutical Supplements in the Treatment of Hypertension," *World Journal of Cardiology* 6, no. 2 (Feb. 26, 2014): 38–66.

23. T. Pentinat et al., "Transgenerational Inheritance of Glucose Intolerance in a Mouse Model of Neonatal Overnutrition," *Endocrinology* 151, no. 12 (Dec. 2010): 5617–23, doi:10.1210/en.2010-0684.

24. G. Kaati et al. "Cardiovascular and Diabetes Mortality Determined by Nutrition during Parents' and Grandparents' Slow Growth Period," *European Journal of Human Genetics* 10 (2002): 682–88.

25. H. Tapp et al., "Nutritional Factors and Gender Influence Age-Related DNA Methylation In the Human Rectal Mucosa," *Aging Cell* (2012), doi:10.1111/acel.12030.

26. J. V. Sanchez-Mut et al., "Promoter Hypermethylation of the Phosphatase DUSP22 Mediates PKA-Dependent TAU Phosphorylation and CREB Activation in Alzheimer's Disease," *Hippocampus* (2014), doi:10.1002/hipo.22245.

27. P. Elwood et al., "Healthy Lifestyles Reduce the Incidence of Chronic Diseases and Dementia: Evidence from the Caerphilly Cohort Study," *PLoS One* (Dec. 2013), doi:10.1371/journal.pone.0081877.

28. D. Ornish et al., "Effect of Comprehensive Lifestyle Changes on Telomerase Activity and Telomere Length in Men with Biopsy-Proven Low-Risk Prostate Cancer: 5-Year Follow-Up of a Descriptive Pilot Study," *Lancet Oncology* 14, no. 11 (Oct. 2013): 1112–20.

29. A. Tiainen et al., "Leukocyte Telomere Length and Its Relation to Food and Nutrient Intake in an Elderly Population," *European Journal of Clinical Nutrition*, 66, no. 12 (Dec. 2012): 1290–94.

30. http://epic.iarc.fr/keyfindings.php.

31. E. Guallar et al., "Enough Is Enough: Stop Wasting Money on Vitamin and Mineral Supplements," *Annals of Internal Medicine* 159, no. 12 (Dec. 17, 2013): 850–51.

32. F. Grodstein et al., "A Randomized Trial of Long-term Multivitamin Supplementation and Cognitive Function in Men: The Physicians' Health Study II," *Annals of Internal Medicine* 159, no. 12 (Dec. 17, 2013): 806–14.

33. J. Walker et al., "Oral Folic Acid and Vitamin B-12 Supplementation to Prevent Cognitive Decline in Community-Dwelling Older Adults with Depressive Symp-

toms—The Beyond Ageing Project: A Randomized Controlled Trial, *American Journal of Clinical Nutrition* 95, no. 1 (Jan. 2012): 194–203.

34. A. D. Smith et al., "Homocysteine-Lowering by B Vitamins Slows the Rate of Accelerated Brain Atrophy in Mild Cognitive Impairment: A Randomized Controlled Trial," *PLoS One* 5, no. 9 (Sept. 2010), doi:10.1371/journal .pone.0012244.

35. B. Small et al., "Nutraceutical Intervention Improves Older Adults' Cognitive Functioning," *Rejuvenation Research*, 17, no. 1 (Feb. 2014): 27–32.

36. G. Douaud et al., "Preventing Alzheimer's Disease-Related Gray Matter Atrophy by B-Vitamin Treatment," *Proceedings of the National Academy of Sciences* 110, no. 23 (June 2013): 9523–28.

37. http://www.sciencedaily.com/releases/2013/11/131104142343.htm.

38. J. Dysken et al., "Effect of Vitamin E and Memantine on Functional Decline in Alzheimer Disease," *JAMA* 311, no. 1 (Jan. 2014): 33–44.

39. J. Sanmukhani et al., "Efficacy and Safety of Curcumin in Major Depressive Disorder: A Randomized Controlled Trial," *Phytotherapy Research* 28, no. 4 (Apr. 2014): 579–85.

40. T. Crook et al., "Effects of Phosphatidylserine in Alzheimer's disease," *Pharmacology Bulletin* 28, no. 1 (1992): 61–66.

41. http://www.greenmedinfo.com/article/alpha-lipoic-acid-anti-inflammatory-and-neuroprotective-treatment-alzheimers.

42. J. Douillard, *The 3-Season Diet* (New York: Harmony Books, 2001).

43. M. Levine et al., "Low Protein Intake Is Associated with a Major Reduction in IGF-1, Cancer, and Overall Mortality in the 65 and Younger but Not Older Population," *Cell Metabolism* 19, no. 3 (2014): 407–17, doi:10.1016 /j.cmet.2014.02.006.

44. http://www.ewg.org/foodnews/summary.php.

45. http://www.edf.org/sites/default/files/1980_pocket_seafood_selector.pdf.

46. S. Weyerer et al., "Current Alcohol Consumption and Its Relationship to Incident Dementia: Results from a 3-Year Follow-Up Study among Primary Care Attenders Aged 75 Years and Older," *Age Ageing* 40 (2011): 456–63.

47. S. Sabia et al. "Alcohol Consumption and Cognitive Decline in Early Old Age," *Neurology* 82 (2014): 332–39.

7. A Youthful Brain Cultivates Curiosity: Key 4

1. J. Rodrigue et al., "Induced Mood and Curiosity," *Cognitive Therapy and Research* 11, no. 1 (1987): 101–6.

2. J. Litman and T. Jimerson, "The Measurement of Curiosity as a Feeling of Deprivation," *Journal of Personality* 82, no. 2 (2004): 147–57.

3. J. E. Joseph, X. Liu, Y. Jiang, D. Lynam, and T. H. Kelly, "Neural Correlates of Emotional Reactivity in Sensation Seeking," *Psychological Science* 20, no. 2 (2008): 215–23.

4. M. Kang et al., "The Hunger for Knowledge: Neural Correlates of Curiosity" (manuscript), Division of Humanities and Social Sciences, California Institute of Technology.

5. T. B. Kashdan and M. F. Steger, "Curiosity and Pathways to Well-Being and Meaning in Life: Traits, States, and Everyday Behaviors," *Motivation and Emotion* 31, no. 3 (2007), 159–73.

6. T. B. Kashdan and P. J. Silvia (2009), "Curiosity and Interest: The Benefits of Thriving on Novelty and Challenge," in S. J. Lopez, ed., *Handbook of Positive Psychology*, 2nd ed. (New York: Oxford University Press).
7. D. C. Park and I. McDonough, "The Dynamic Aging Mind: Revelations from Functional Neuroimaging Research," *Perspectives in Psychological Science* 8 (2013): 62–67.
8. L. Shlain, *Art & Physics: Parallel Visions in Space, Time and Light* (New York: Harper Perennial, 1991).
9. Shlain, ibid., p. 16.
10. L. Carroll, *Alice's Adventures In Wonderland*, chap. 1, "Down the Rabbit Hole" (New York: Bantam Dell, 1981; first published 1865).
11. W. Pisula et al., "Comparative Psychology as Unified Psychology: The Case of Curiosity and Other Novelty-Related Behavior," *Review of General Psychology* 17, no. 2 (2013): 224–29.
12. J. Litman, "Curiosity and the Pleasures of Learning: Wanting and Liking New Information," *Cognition and Emotion* 19, no. 6 (2005): 793–814.
13. A. Gosline, "Bored to death: Chronically Bored People Exhibit Higher Risk-Taking Behavior," *Scientific American*, Feb. 26, 2007, www.sciam.com/article.cfm?id=bored—find-something-to-live-for.
14. C. Yarnal and X. Qian, "Older-Adult Playfulness: An Innovative Construct and Measurement for Healthy Aging Research," *American Journal of Play* 4, no. 1 (2011): 52–79.
15. Robert Frost, "The Road Not Taken" (poem), *Mountain Interval* (New York: Henry Holt, 1915).

8. A Youthful Brain Stays Flexible: Key 5

1. E. Goldberg, *The Wisdom Paradox* (New York: Gotham Books, 2005).
2. C. Herzog et al., "Enrichment Effects on Adult Cognitive Development," *Psychological Science in the Public Interest* 9, no. 1 (2008): 1–65.
3. B. Chanowitz and E. Langer, "Premature Cognitive Commitment," *Journal of Personality and Social Psychology* 41, no. 6 (1981): 51–63.
4. E. Langer, *Mindfulness* (New York: Da Capo Press, 1989).
5. Bob Greene, *20 Years Younger* (New York: Little, Brown, 2012).
6. C. Coppens et al. (2010). "Coping Styles and Behavioural Flexibility: Towards Underlying Mechanisms," *Philosophical Transactions of the Royal Society* 365, no. 1560 (2015): 4021–28.
7. D. Kahneman, *Thinking, Fast and Slow* (New York: Farrar, Straus and Giroux, 2011).
8. J. Hawley, *The Bhagavad Gita: A Walkthrough for Westerners* (San Francisco: New World Library, 2001).
9. M. Merzenich, *Soft-Wired*, 2nd ed. (San Francisco: Parnassus Publishing, 2013).
10. D. Durstewitz et al. "Abrupt Transitions between Prefrontal Neural Ensemble States Accompany Behavioral Transitions during Rule Learning," *Neuron* 66 (2010): 438–48.
11. S. Floresco, "Prefrontal Dopamine and Behavioral Flexibility," *Frontiers in Neuroscience* 7, no. 62 (2013).
12. G. Buzsáki, *Rhythms of the Brain* (New York: Oxford University Press, 2006).
13. K. Druck, *The Real Rules of Life: Balancing Life's Terms with Your Own* (New York: Hay House Publishing, 2012), p. vxi.

14. D. Zabelina and M. Beeman, "Short-Term Attentional Perseveration Associated with Real-Life Creative Achievement," *Frontiers in Psychology* 4 (2013): 191.
15. Ibid.
16. A. S. Griffin, D. Guez, F. Lermite, and M. Patience, "Tracking Changing Environments: Innovators Are Fast, but Not Flexible Learners," *PLoS ONE* 8, no.12 (2013): e84907, doi10.1371/journal.pone.0084907.
17. P. Greenwood, *Nurturing the Older Brain and Mind* (Cambridge, MA: MIT Press, 2012).
18. J. Singer, *Memories that Matter* (Oakland, CA: New Harbinger Publications, 2005).

9. A Youthful Brain Is Optimistic: Key 6

1. D. Hecht, "The Neural Basis of Optimism and Pessimism," *Experimental Neurobiology* 22, no. 3 (2013): 173–99.
2. A. Reading, *Hope and Despair: How Perceptions of the Future Shape Human Behavior* (Baltimore: The Johns Hopkins University Press, 2004), 3.
3. L. Abramson, M. Seligman, and J. Teasdale, "Learned Helplessness in Humans: Critique and Reformulation," *Journal of Abnormal Psychology* 87, no. 1 (1978): 49–74.
4. T. Sharot et al., "Dopamine Enhances Expectation of Pleasure in Humans," *Current Biology* (2009), doi:10.1016/j.cub.2009.10.025.
5. T. Sharot, C. Korn, and R. J. Dolan, "How Unrealistic Optimism Is Maintained in the Face of Reality," *Nature Neuroscience* 14 (2011): 1475–79.
6. C. Moutsiana, N. Garrett, R. C. Clarke, R. B. Lotto, S. J. Blakemore, and T. Sharot, "Human Development of the Ability to Learn from Bad News, *Proceedings of the National Academy of Sciences* 110, no. 41(2013): 16396–401.
7. R. Hanson and R. Mendius, *Buddha's Brain: Practical Neuroscience of Happiness, Love and Wisdom* (Oakland, CA: New Harbinger Publications, 2009).
8. C. Korn, T. Sharot, H. Walter, H. R. Heekeren, and R. J. Dolan, "Depression Is Related to an Absence of Optimistically Biased Belief Updating about Future Life Events," *Psychological Medicine* 44 (2014): 579–92.
9. R. Chowdhury, T. Sharot, T. Wolfe, E. Düzel, and R. J. Dolan, "Optimistic Update Bias Increases in Older Age," *Psychological Medicine* 4 (2013): 1–10.
10. M. Gallagher, S. Lopez, and S. Pressman, "Optimism Is Universal: Exploring the Presence and Benefits of Optimism in a Representative Sample of the World," *Journal of Personality* 81, no. 5 (2013): 429–40.
11. R. Chowdhury, T. Sharot, T. Wolfe, E. Düzel, and R. J. Dolan, "Optimistic Update Bias Increases in Older Age."
12. S. H. Kim, B. Cornwell, and S. E. Kim, "Individual Differences in Emotion Regulation and Hemispheric Metabolic Asymmetry," *Biological Psychology* 89 (2012): 382–86.
13. R. Davidson, "Affective Neuroscience and Psychophysiology: Toward a Synthesis," *Psychophysiology* 40, no. 5 (2003): 655–65.
14. K. Kakolewski et al., "Laterality Word Valence, and Visual Attention: A Comparison of Depressed and Non-Depressed Individuals," *International Journal of Psychophysiology* 34 (1999): 283–92.
15. M. Seligman, *Learned Optimism: How to Change Your Mind and Your Life,* 2nd ed. (New York: Pocket Books, 1998).

16. M. Yapko, *Depression Is Contagious* (New York: Free Press, 2009).
17. A. Leaver, J. Van Lare, B. Zielinski, A. Halpern, and J. Rauschecker, "Brain Activation during Anticipation of Sound Sequences," *Journal of Neuroscience* 29, no. 8 (2009), 2477, doi:10.1523/JNEUROSCI.4921-08.2009.
18. K. Walker and A. King, "Auditory Neuroscience: Temporal Anticipation Enhances Cortical Processing," *Current Biology* 12:21, no. 7 (2011), R251-3, doi:10.1016/j.cub.2011.02.022.
19. R. Sapolsky, "Are Humans Just Another Primate?" Pritzker Lecture, California Academy of Sciences, Feb. 15, 2011: retrieved Apr. 20, 2014, from http://video .calacademy.org/details/349.
20. Gilbert, P., *The Compassionate Mind* (Oakland, CA: New Harbinger Publications, 2009).

10. A Youthful Brain Is Empathic: Key 7

1. J. Crabtree, "Agnes the Ageing Suit," *FT Magazine*, July 22, 2011: retrieved May 6, 2014, from www.ft.com/cms/s/2/1fed1eee-b34b-11e0-9af2-00144feabdc0 .html.
2. P. Bailey and J. Henry, "Growing Less Empathic with Age: Disinhibition of the Self-Perspective," *Journal of Gerontology* 63B, no. 4 (2008): 19–26.
3. G. Labouvie-Vief et al., "Dynamic Emotion-Cognition Interactions in Development: Arousal, Stress, and the Processing of Affect," in *Aging and Cognition*, ed. H. B. Bosworth and C. Hertzog (Washington, DC: American Psychological Association, 2009).
4. W. Cannon, "The James-Lange Theory of Emotions: A Critical Examination and an Alternative Theory," *The American Journal of Psychology* 39 (1927): 106–24.
5. G. Rizzolatti et al., "Functional Organization of Inferior Area 6 in the Macaque Monkey: Area 5 and the Control of Distal Movements," *Experimental Brain Research* 71 (1998): 491–507.
6. V. Gallese and A. Goldman, "Mirror Neurons and the Stimulation Theory of Mind-Reading," *Trends in Cognitive Sciences* 2 (1998): 493–501.
7. T. Insel and L. Young, "The Neurobiology of Attachment," *Nature Reviews: Neuroscience* 2 (2001): 129–36.
8. A. Schore, "Effects of a Secure Attachment Relationship on Right Brain Development, Affect Regulation and Infant Mental Health," *Infant Mental Health Journal* 1–2 (2001): 7–66.
9. A. Schore, "Attachment and Regulation of the Right Brain," *Attachment and Human Development* 2, no. 1 (2000): 23–47.
10. A. Schore, "Paradigm Shift: The Right Brain and the Relational Unconscious," *American Psychological Association*, invited speaker, lecture conducted for Plenary Session at the American Psychological Association Annual Convention, Toronto, Canada, Aug. 8, 2009.
11. A. Schore, "Effects of a Secure Attachment Relationship."
12. A. Schore, "Attachment and Regulation of the Right Brain."
13. A. Schore, "Paradigm Shift."
14. W. A. Collins and L. A. Sroufe, "Capacity for Intimate Relationships: A Developmental Construction," in W. Furman, B. B. Brown, and C. Feiring, eds., *The Development of Romantic Relationships in Adolescence* (New York: Cambridge University Press, 1999).

15. M. Solomon, "Emotion in Romantic Partners: Intimacy Found, Intimacy Lost, Intimacy Reclaimed," in D. Fosha, D. Siegel, and M. Solomon, eds., *The Healing Power of Emotion: Affective Neuroscience, Development and Clinical Practice* (New York: W. W. Norton, 2009).

16. M. Lucas, *Rewire Your Brain for Love: Creating Vibrant Relationships Using the Science of Mindfulness* (Carlsbad, CA: Hay House Publishing, 2012).

17. J. Sze et al., "Greater Emotional Empathy and Prosocial Behavior in Late Life," *Emotion* 12, no. 5 (2012): 1129–40.

18. R. Levenson, "Emotion and Emotion Regulation," in *Changing Emotions*, ed. D. Hermans, B. Rimé, and B. Mesquita (New York: Psychology Press, 2013), 105–12.

19. G. Labouvie-Vief, *Psyche and Eros: Mind and Gender in The Life Course* (New York: Cambridge University Press, 1995).

20. B. Kok et al., "How Positive Emotions Build Physical Health: Perceived Positive Social Connections Account for Upward Spiral between Positive Emotions and Vagal Tone," *Psychological Science* 24, no. 7 (2013): 1123–32.

21. C. D. Batson et al., eds., "Empathy and Altruism," *Oxford Handbook of Positive Psychology,* 2nd ed. (New York: Oxford University Press, 2009).

22. B. Schwartz, *Rippling: How Social Entrepreneurs Spread Innovation throughout the World* (New York: John Wiley & Sons, 2012).

23. T. Hacker, "Building Empathy Builds Society," *The Seattle Times,* Jan. 28, 2013.

24. J. Eakin, *Living Autobiographically: How We Create Identity in Narrative* (Ithaca: Cornell University Press, 2008).

25. P. Eriksson and L. Wallin, "Functional Consequences of Stress-Related Suppression of Adult Hippocampal Neurogenesis: A Novel Hypothesis on the Neurobiology of Burnout," *Acta Neurologica Scandinavia* 110, no. 5 (2004): 275–80.

26. J. D. Bremner, *Does Stress Damage the Brain?* (New York: W. W. Norton & Co., 2002).

27. M. Crockett et al., "Serotonin Selectively Influences Moral Judgment and Behavior through Effects on Harm Aversion," Proceedings of The National Academy of Sciences 107, no. 40 (2010), retrieved May 19, 2014, doi:10.1073/pnas.1009396107.

28. J. T. Cacioppo et al., "Social Neuroscience: Progress and Implications for Mental Health," *Perspectives on Psychological Science* 2, no. 2 (2007): 99–123.

29. C. Yarnal and X. Qian, "Older-Adult playfulness: An Innovative Construct and Measurement for Healthy Aging Research," *American Journal of Play* 4, no. 1 (2011): 52–78.

30. E. Y. Cornwell and L. J. Waite, "Social Disconnectedness, Perceived Isolation, and Health among Older Adults," *Journal of Health and Social Behavior* 50, no. 1 (2009): 31–48.

31. T. Schmid, *Promoting Health through Creativity: For Professionals in Health, Arts and Education* (London, England: Whurr Publishers Ltd., 2005).

11. A Youthful Brain Is Well Connected: Key 8

1. C. Pasquaretta et al., "Social Networks in Primates: Smart and Tolerant Species Have More Efficient Networks," *Scientific Reports* 4, Article number 7600 (Dec. 2014), doi:10.1038/srep07600.

2. K. M. Kendrick, "The Neurobiology of Social Bonds," *Journal of Neuroendocrinology* 16, no. 12 (Dec 2004): 1007–8.

3. P. L. Wachtel, *Relational Therapy and the Practice of Psychotherapy* (New York: Guilford Publishing, 2008).

4. L. Cozolino, *The Neuroscience of Human Relationships: Attachment and the Developing Social Brain* (New York: W.W. Norton, 2006).

5. D. Wallin, *Attachment in Psychotherapy* (New York: Guilford Publishing, 2007), 101.

6. L. M. Matire and M. M. Franks, "The Role of Social Networks in Adult Health: Introduction to the Special Issue," *Health Psychology* 33, no. 6 (2014), 501–4.

7. J. K. Kiecolt-Glaser and T. L. Newton, "Marriage and Health: His and Hers," *Psychological Bulletin* 127 (2001): 472–503.

8. M. M. Franks et al., "I Will If You Will: Similarity in Health Behavior Change of Married Partners," *Health Education and Behavior* 39 (2012): 324–31.

9. R. S. Sneed, and S. Cohen, "Negative Social Interactions and Incident Hypertension among Older Adults," *Health Psychology* 33 (2014): 554–65.

10. S. T. Cheng et al., "Physical and Social Activities Mediate the Associations between Social Network Types and Ventilator Function in Chinese Older Adults," *Health Psychology* 33 (2014): 524–34.

11. J. Hollis, *The Eden Project: In Search of the Magical Other* (Toronto: Inner City Books, 1998), 13.

12. C. J. Jung, "Commentary on 'The Secret of the Golden Flower,'" in *Collected Works*, vol. 13, *Alchemical Studies* (UK: Routledge & Kegan Paul, 1967), 47–48.

13. U.S. Department of Health and Human Services, "Prevention Makes Common 'Cents'": http://aspe.hhs.gov/health/prevention/prevention.pdf (2003).

14. A. Golay et al., "Motivating for Change: A New Approach," *Service of Therapeutic Education for Chronic Diseases*, Didactic Science Laboratory, Geneva, Switzerland, 2012.

15. N. L. Kerr and C. M. Kaufman-Gililand, "Communication, Commitment, and Cooperation in Social Dilemma," *Journal of Personality and Social Psychology* 66, no. 3 (1994): 513–29.

16. K. M. Brethel-Haurwitz and A. A. Marsh, Geographical Differences in Subjective Well-Being Predict Extraordinary Altruism, *Psychological Science* 25, no. 3 (2014): 762–71.

17. V. E. Frankl, *The Unheard Cry for Meaning: Psychotherapy and Humanism* (New York: Simon & Schuster, 1978).

18. M. Freedman, *Encore: Finding Work That Matters in the Second Half of Life* (New York: Perseus Books Group, 2007).

19. W. Muller, *How, Then, Shall We Live?* (New York: Bantam, 1996).

20. M. Buber, *I and Thou* (New York: Charles Scribner's Sons, 1970).

21. E. Renehan et al., "Healthy Aging Literature Review," *National Ageing Research Institute* and *Council on the Ageing*, 2012, prepared for the Victoria, Australia, Department of Health, www.health.vic.gov.au/agedcare.

22. B. Cornwell, E. O. Laumann, and L. P. Schumm, "The Social Connectedness of Older Adults: A National Profile," *American Sociological Review* 73, no. 2 (2008): 185–203.

23. Quoted from "Addressing Isolation among Older Adults: The Role of Social Connectedness in Healthy Aging," report of The National Council on Aging, 2014, www.illuminage.com/webinars/presentations/webinar-052214.pdf.

24. C. A. Emlet and J. T. Moceri, "The Importance of Social Connectedness in Building Age-Friendly Communities," *Journal of Aging Research* 2012, article ID 173247, 9 pages, http://dx.doi.org/10.1155/2012/173247.

25. V. Toepoel, "Aging, Leisure, and Social Connectedness: How Could Leisure Help Reduce Social Isolation of Older People?" *Social Indicators Research* 113 (2013): 355–72.

26. D. Whyte, *Everything Is Waiting for You* (Langley, WA: Many Rivers Press, 2003).

12. A Youthful Brain Is Authentic: Key 9

1. http://rabbidavidkominsky.com/tag/zusya/. Used with permission.

2. P. Palmer, *Let Your Life Speak: Listening to the Voice of Vocation* (New York: John Wiley & Sons, 2000).

3. Ibid.

4. P. Nelson, *There's A Hole in My Sidewalk* (Hillsboro, OR: Beyond Words, 1993).

5. M. Oliver, "When Death Comes," *New and Selected Poems* (Boston: Beacon Press, 2004).

6. S. Haldeman-Martz, ed., *If I Had My Life to Live Over, I Would Pick More Daisies* (Watsonville, CA: Papier-Mache Press, 2010).

7. W. Muller, *A Life of Being, Having, and Doing Enough* (New York: Harmony, 2011).

About the Authors

Henry Emmons, MD, is a psychiatrist who integrates mind-body and natural therapies, mindfulness teachings, and compassion and insight into his clinical work. His career has been animated by the desire to develop more integrative (holistic) approaches for such common mental health problems as depression and anxiety. He practices with Partners in Resilience, where they offer Pathways to Resilience, a program that integrates the best of movement, nutrition, natural therapies, and the psychology of mindfulness to help restore resilience and rediscover joy.

Dr. Emmons is a sought-after presenter and a respected consultant on such topics as integrating natural and mindfulness therapies in psychiatry, the interface between spirituality and mental health, and personal and professional renewal. He has developed several transformational programs, including A Year of Living Mindfully and The Inner Life of Healers through the University of Minnesota's Center for Spirituality and Healing; and Resilience Training at the Penny George Institute for Health and Healing. He is also a founding board member of the International Network for Integrative Mental Health.

He is the author of three earlier books: *The Chemistry of Joy: A Three-Step Program for Overcoming Depression Through Western Science and Eastern Wisdom* (Simon & Schuster, 2005); *The Chemistry of Calm: A Powerful, Drug-Free Plan to Quiet Your Fears and Over-*

come Your Anxiety (Simon & Schuster, 2010); and *The Chemistry of Joy Workbook: Overcoming Depression Using the Best of Brain Science, Nutrition, and the Psychology of Mindfulness* (New Harbinger, 2012).

David Alter, PhD, is a clinical health and neuropsychologist. He is the cofounder of Partners in Healing of Minneapolis, an integrative medicine center where he conducts his clinical practice. His holistic treatment approach helps clients to deepen their sense of life's meaning and purpose, to create more fulfilling lives, and to return to health when suffering from chronic illness conditions affecting their mind and body. He also works with couples to help them gain the emotional and physical health benefits of creating intimately interconnected lives.

He has developed several innovative, group-based programs—including The Conscious Living Program, for individuals suffering with chronic pain, and Getting to the Guts of What Matters, for individuals suffering from digestive illnesses—which combine engaged learning and active skill-building practices to help put people back in charge of their lives. His integrative, neuroscience-based approach, when coupled with practices drawn from ancient wisdom traditions, helps people go beyond symptom relief to develop skills and practices enabling them to express their best and highest selves throughout their lives.

Dr. Alter is an engaging and sought-after speaker and teacher at local, national, and international conferences, and trainings covering a wide range of topics specifically tailored to each audience's needs. He also offers presentations, workshops, retreats, and seminars to professional, faith-based, patient, and general audiences. His trainings enable participants to access and activate their mind-body-spirit connections to bring greater happiness and satisfaction into their lives and into the lives of others.

Both authors can be contacted at: www.StayingSharp.org.